CURRENT TOPICS IN IMMUNOLOGY

General editor: Professor John Turk

No. 7 Immunology of the Rheumatic Diseases

For our families, for their patience.
With love and thanks

Immunology of the Rheumatic Diseases
Aspects of Autoimmunity

R. N. Maini, M.R.C.P.

Consultant Rheumatologist to Charing Cross Hospital, London;
Deputy Head, Clinical Research Division, Kennedy Institute of
Rheumatology, London

D. N. Glass, M.R.C.P.

Arthritis and Rheumatism Council Research Fellow at Robert B. Brigham
Hospital, Boston; formerly Senior Registrar, Charing Cross Hospital,
and Maynard-Jenour Fellow at the Kennedy Institute of Rheumatology, London

J. T. Scott, M.D., F.R.C.P.

Consultant Physician to Charing Cross Hospital, London;
Deputy Director and Head of Clinical Research Division,
Kennedy Institute of Rheumatology, London

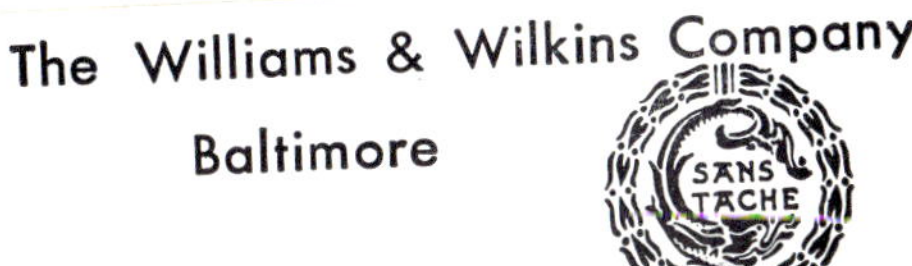

First published 1977
by Edward Arnold (Publishers) Ltd.
25 Hill Street, London W1X 8LL

ISBN: 0 7131 4279 0

Set in 10 on 11pt Imprint at Western Printing Services Ltd.
Reproduced and printed by photolithography and bound
in Great Britain at The Pitman Press, Bath

General Preface to Series

The impact of immunological thought on medical practice has been increasing at a steady rate now for nearly twenty years. There appear to be very few fields to which the immunologist cannot contribute. Initially the immunological approach was limited to assistance in diagnosis and in sera and vaccine production. New approaches in the field of therapy are not only in the use of vaccines, sera and immunosuppressive agents, but also in the more rational use of conventional therapeutic agents. Immunological knowledge is especially necessary in the field of tumour therapy, particularly in the balanced use of surgery and radiotherapy. Moreover, immunological knowledge in other fields has allowed us to understand more readily the mechanisms whereby a single aetiological agent can produce a wide range of different clinical manifestations. Different disease patterns occur depending on the nature of the immunological reaction causing tissue damage. A completely different symptom complex from reactions involving soluble immune complexes reacting with the complement cascade will be found in those involving the reaction of specifically sensitized lymphocytes with antigen as part of a cell-mediated or delayed hypersensitivity reaction.

As a massive amount of new scientific material accumulates in this field, the clinician is frequently left behind and perplexed. Each year a new scientific journal is published specializing in fields as diverse as immunogenetics, immunochemistry or immunological techniques. We have journals emanating from continents as well as countries. The wealth of material is often bewildering. Simple textbooks of immunology are often too simple, whereas review articles may be too complicated for the specialist physician or surgeon who wants a treatise on those aspects of the subject particularly relevant to his own field of interest. It is hoped that this series will fulfil some of these needs by giving comparatively short reviews that will lay emphasis on immunological subjects which should appeal to both clinicians and those working in clinical laboratories. The aim is to provide the busy clinician in a particular field of medicine with a short volume relevant to his practice written by a specialist. It should introduce the reader to the immunological approach to his subject and indicate how modern immunological thought might influence his day-to-day work in the wards or clinical laboratory.

JOHN TURK

The Royal College of Surgeons of England
London

Preface

It is now nearly thirty years since three independent and almost simultaneous observations—the discovery of rheumatoid factor, the description of the LE cell phenomenon, and the dramatic effect of cortisone on rheumatoid arthritis—heralded the present era in which rheumatic diseases have come to occupy a pre-eminent place in the rapidly developing science of clinical immunology.

This book is intended mainly for clinicians who are interested in discovering how immunological concepts have contributed to our understanding of the pathogenesis of certain rheumatic diseases, and how immunological methods have been applied to the clinical management of patients. Rheumatic diseases involve primarily the joints and locomotor structures but they also manifest systemic features and involvement of other organs, so that rheumatology is now recognized as an integral branch of internal medicine. It is hoped that our readership will include all those who want to enlarge their knowledge about the application of immunology to clinical medicine, in particular practising rheumatologists, immunologists, post-graduate students, physicians, pathologists and research workers.

The first section of the book begins with an account and analysis of the biology of the immune response and its relevance to protective immunity, tolerance, hypersensitivity and the cellular basis of autoimmunity. The following two chapters discuss the relationship of immune responses to tissue injury and the significance of antibodies and cell-mediated reactions against a large variety of autoantigens. The final chapter of this section is intended to familiarize clinicians with immunological methods and their application to investigative rheumatology.

Section B is essentially concerned with phenomenology. Diseases such as rheumatoid arthritis and systemic lupus erythematosus have been chosen to demonstrate in some detail the application of immunological studies to their clinical manifestations. Sjögren's syndrome is chosen because of its close relationship to both rheumatoid arthritis and systemic lupus erythematosus, and because it perhaps exemplifies the importance of impaired immunological surveillance in the pathogenesis of the disease itself and accompanying predisposition to malignancy. In contrast to these disorders, in which immune complexes have been implicated as an important pathogenetic mechanism, cellular immunity appears to be of primary significance in polymyositis. In myasthenia gravis the pathological basis of impaired neuromuscular transmission remains unsolved but some interesting ideas have been put forward about the hormonal role of the thymus gland and the possibility of autoantibodies directed against cell membrane receptors. Relapsing polychondritis has been chosen because immunological responses to connective tissue components (antigenic sites in matrix) make it a possible contender as the only true example of 'autoallergic connective tissue disease'. A chapter on infections in arthritis deals with the ways in which infection may involve joints and provides an insight into possible interactions between organisms, the immune response and joint inflammation. Vasculitis mediated by immune complexes and possibly by cellular mechanisms is, in a sense, central to the pathology of inflammation observed in a variety of rheumatic diseases. Some of the more recent investigations summarized in this chapter suggest unifying pathogenetic concepts, but many interesting questions remain unanswered; for example, the reason why different blood vessels and sites of localization are observed in well recognized clinical syndromes. The final chapter in this section considers briefly the therapeutic implications of immunological pathogenesis, particularly the use of immunosuppressive agents. Although a good theoretical case can be made for such treatment, the evidence for their value in some of the rheumatic diseases is controversial.

In the last section the possibility is considered that these diseases evolve against a background of genetic susceptibility. In fact, epidemiological evidence for such predisposition is conclusive only for ankylosing spondylitis and, to a certain extent, systemic lupus erythematosus. The possibility that diseases result from deficiency of genetically controlled capacity to synthesize immunoglobulin or complement on the one hand, and development of antigen-specific immune responses peculiar to the individual, on the other, is discussed in this section.

We should like to acknowledge the help of Miss Lindsay Roffe of the Kennedy Institute in drawing the line diagrams and Dr David Woodrow, Professor John Sloper and Dr David Yates of Charing Cross Hospital for Figures 5.2 and 6.1. A word of grateful thanks is also expressed to our secretaries Miss Teresa Kearney and Mrs Mary Wheeler who have patiently typed the numerous drafts and produced the final version of this book without protest and at great speed, and to Marianne Maini for her help with proof reading.

R.N.M.
D.N.G.

London 1976   J.T.S.

Contents

General Preface to Series   v

Preface   vii

Section A.
Aspects of Basic Immunology, Tissue Damage, Autoimmunity and Methods of Study

1 Biological Aspects of the Immune Response   3

Introduction
Lymphocytes and macrophages in induction of immune responses and
    tolerance
    Thymus-dependent T lymphocytes
    B lymphocytes
    Macrophages
Hypersensitivity reactions to antigens
    Type I reactions
    Type II reactions
    Type III reactions
    Type IV reactions
Genetic control of immune response and complement metabolism
Cellular mechanisms of autoimmunity
    Bypass of T cell intolerance
    Intrinsic abnormalities of cellular and humoral immunity
    Loss of suppressor T cell function

2 Mechanisms of Tissue Injury   13

Pathophysiology of tissue damage
    Vascular damage
    Cellular damage
    Matrix damage
Immune complexes and tissue damage
    Formation and deposition of immune complexes
    Pathogenesis of tissue injury
    Role of complement
    Role of polymorphonuclear neutrophils and macrophages
Cell-mediated tissue injury
    Pathogenesis
    Mechanisms of cell-mediated cytotoxicity
    Additional forms of cell-mediated tissue injury

3 Immune Reactions to Autoantigens   23

Autoantibodies
    Rheumatoid factors

        Nature and occurrence
        Heterogeneity
        IgM and IgG rheumatoid factors
        Clinical significance
     Other antiglobulin factors
     Antibodies to chondrocytes
     Antibodies to proteoglycans
     Antibodies to collagen
     Anti-nuclear antibodies
        Immunofluorescent tests
        Antibody to defined nuclear and cytoplasmic antigens
        Heterogeneity
  Cellular immunity to autoantigens
     Reactions to IgG
     Reactions to synovial cells
     Reactions to other antigens

4 Immunological Methods   **38**

     Studies on fresh tissues
        Source of material
        Microscopy
     Immunochemistry of tissue fluids and eluates
     Tissue culture
     Complement
     Measurement of circulating immune complexes
     Tests of cellular immunity
        Sheep erythrocyte rosettes
        Antisera against T cells
        Surface immunoglobulin
        Surface complement (C3) receptor
        Surface Fc receptor
        Glass adherence
        Nylon-fibre and antibody-coated columns
        Staining of cytoplasm for enzymes
        Cell-mediated cytotoxicity
        Delayed hypersensitivity
        Lymphocyte transformation
        Lymphokine production

Section B.
Applied Immunology and Connective Tissue Diseases

5 Rheumatoid Arthritis   **53**

     Immunopathology of joint disease
     The synovium: an ectopic lymphoid organ
     Immune complexes in synovial membrane and fluid

Circulating immune complexes and vasculitis
Nodules
Complement
Rheumatoid factors
Relative importance of humoral and cellular immunity in pathogenesis
Lymphocytes in synovial membrane and fluid
Lymphocyte subpopulations in peripheral blood
Immune status
Immune status in juvenile rheumatoid arthritis
Immune reactions to infective agents

6 Systemic Lupus Erythematosus   71

Introduction
Joint disease
Kidney
Central nervous system
Skin manifestations
Vascular disease
Liver
Lungs
Haematological abnormalities
Autoimmune serological phenomena
Immune complexes and complement
Lymphocyte subpopulations
Immune status
Infective aetiological theory
Relationship between chronic discoid and systemic lupus erythematosus
Drug-induced lupus erythematosus

7 Sjögren's Syndrome   89

Clinical features
Immunopathology
Autoantibodies
Cell-mediated immunity
   Lymphocyte function
   Enumeration of peripheral lymphocyte populations
Relationship to lymphoproliferative disorders

8 Polymyositis and Myasthenia Gravis   94

Introduction
Clinicopathological features
   Type α
   Type β
   Type γ
Immunology of polymyositis
   Association with immunodeficiency and neoplastic disease

Immunology of myasthenia gravis
   Thymus and anti-skeletal muscle antibodies
   Anti-nuclear, lymphocytotoxic and anti-receptor antibodies
   Thymic factors
   Cellular immunity

9 Relapsing Polychondritis   **101**

10 Infections and Arthritis   **103**

Introduction
Classification
Rheumatic fever
Meningococcal arthritis
Arthritis associated with hepatitis B infection

11 Vasculitis and Polyarteritis Nodosa   **112**

Vasculitis: definition; classification; pathogenesis
Vasculitis in rheumatoid arthritis
Vasculitis in other connective tissue diseases
Polyarteritis nodosa
Giant cell (temporal) arteritis
Pulseless disease
Wegener's granulomatosis
Behcet's syndrome
Henoch–Schönlein purpura

12 Therapeutic Implications   **119**

Immunosuppression
Cytostatic drugs in connective tissue diseases
   Rheumatoid arthritis
   Systemic lupus erythematosus
   Other diseases
Complications of cytostatic drug therapy
Immunostimulation or immunorestoration

**Section C.
Interrelationships between Genetic Factors, Rheumatic Diseases and
Immune Responses**

**13 Genetic Factors, Immune Response, Complement Deficiency
and Susceptibility to Inflammatory Rheumatic Diseases**   **129**

Introduction
Epidemiology and genetic predisposition
Genetic control of the non-antigen-specific immune response and
   rheumatic disease
   Immunoglobulin deficiency
   Complement component deficiencies

Markers for possible antigen-specific immune response genes and
   rheumatic disease
   HL-A-27 spondylitis
   Other rheumatic diseases
Conclusions

Appendix   139
   New and previous terminologies for major histocompatibility
      region antigens

Index   141

Section A

Aspects of Basic Immunology,
Tissue Damage, Autoimmunity and Methods
of Study

1

Biological Aspects of the Immune Response

Introduction

Numerous changes indicating involvement of immunological responses are observed in some of the rheumatic diseases, particularly the inflammatory disorders of connective tissue such as rheumatoid arthritis and systemic lupus erythematosus. These changes can be defined in terms of cellular and humoral immunological events which are believed to result from the interaction of the lymphoreticular system with antigen. The ensuing reactions evolve around: (1) cells derived from a lymphocyte lineage or related to macrophages; and (2) humoral factors such as antibody and other molecular products originating from these cells. These phenomena have been investigated and documented in tissues and fluids most readily available, which in patients with rheumatic diseases has in practice meant investigating extracellular fluids, such as blood and synovial fluid, and tissues obtained by biopsy, surgery or autopsy. Many of our ideas about immunological responses in rheumatic diseases have also been obtained from animal models.

A study of immune mechanisms in connective tissue diseases is of fundamental importance in understanding the emergence of autoimmune reactions frequently observed in these diseases, and the mediation of various clinicopathological features. Evidence from experimental studies has drawn attention to the central importance of cells belonging to the lymphocyte and macrophage lineage which are intimately concerned with the development of immune responses upon challenge with antigen. Of equal importance is our increasing understanding of the cellular and chemical basis of immunological unresponsiveness (tolerance), which, as postulated by Burnet (1959) is highly selective and allows discrimination by the immune system between 'self' and 'non-self'. Lymphocytes, however, are a heterogeneous cell population in terms of their developmental origins, structure, surface characteristics and diversity of function. Further, their function is determined by complicated patterns of interaction with antigens; cell division; passage via blood and lymphatic channels through lymphoid tissues, thymus, bone marrow and gut; and by interaction between subpopulations of lymphocytes themselves and with other cells, particularly macrophages. Any unitary concept to explain a basic derangement in disease is at risk of being too naïve.

Many types of defect are possible, and numerous current hypotheses are some-times contradictory and hard to reconcile. Nevertheless, we are now in a position to define at least a hypothetical model for the development of immune responses and tolerance to antigens, and to see whether the predictions prove to be of value in understanding the immunological pathogenesis of rheumatic diseases.

Lymphocytes and macrophages in induction of immune responses and tolerance

Introduction of antigen under appropriate conditions either stimulates an immune response or leads to an immunologically unresponsive state (tolerance) which is antigen-specific. At least two distinct lymphocyte populations (in addition to macrophages) are concerned with the development of the immune response (see Roitt *et al.*, 1969) and tolerance in a number of ways.

THYMUS-DEPENDENT T LYMPHOCYTES

Thymus-dependent T lymphocytes are responsible for cell-mediated immunity. Interaction of antigen with sensitized T cells leads to activation of metabolic processes of the cell, increased DNA synthesis, cellular enlargement, and mitosis. These cells operate both by direct contact with other cells and by synthesizing and releasing mediators of cellular immunity, collectively termed 'lymphokines'. They are responsible for: (1) surveillance against tumours and infections; (2) graft rejection; they also (3) participate in the synthesis of antibody in response to most antigens ('helper' effect).

B LYMPHOCYTES

B lymphocytes (thus termed because of their origin in the bursa of Fabricius in the fowl) are the precursors of cells which will synthesize antibody. B cells respond to some antigens independently of T cells, possibly with the involve-ment of macrophages (in which case IgM antibody is usually exclusively pro-duced), but generally require the 'helper' effects of antigen-stimulated T cells.

While administration of antigen normally produces an immunological response, Dresser and Mitchison (1968) have shown that its introduction in certain circumstances (e.g. repeated very low doses) induces T cell tolerance so that B cells remain in a dormant state but under special circumstances are capable of activation; or T and B cell tolerance in which neither T nor B cells respond to antigen (e.g. by appropriate administration of very high doses) (reviewed by Weigle, 1973). Such circumstances were regarded by Allison (1971) and Weigle (1973) as being accountable for tolerance to soluble autoantigens, a postulate that does not entirely support Burnet's original concept of unrespon-siveness due to elimination or seclusion of clones of immunocompetent cells during fetal or infantile life. The current concept of unresponsiveness to auto-antigens is thus complex and the demonstration of B cells reactive against certain autoantigens lends support to the T cell tolerance mechanism. In accordance with this notion, T cell tolerance can be overcome, or bypassed, leading to auto-immunity (i.e. a response to self antigens). The existence of a T cell suppressive effect, inhibiting B cell functional proliferation, has also been proposed, and it has been suggested that these T 'suppressor cells' are important as a second line of defence in controlling the emergence of autoimmunity should low dose T cell tolerance be overcome (Allison *et al.*, 1971). These mechanisms are discussed more fully in the last part of this chapter.

MACROPHAGES

Macrophages are intimately involved in interactions of T and B cells with antigens, and appear to be important in the production of antibody. It has been suggested that they may process antigen and present it in a highly immuno-genic form to B lymphocytes (Unanue, 1972); that they co-operate with T cells in generating a chemical which activates complement, thus providing an im-portant signal for B cell activation (Dukor *et al.*, 1974); that T cell activation by antigen releases a factor which attaches itself to the surface of macrophages, and regulates B cell function (Feldmann and Nossal, 1972); or, as suggested by Ada and Parish (1968), that they are involved in immune stimulation or tolerance depending on the concentration of antigen on the surface of the macrophages and their proximity to B cells in lymphoid organs.

Macrophages, as phagocytic cells, play an important part in immune-complex clearance (involving binding to surface receptors for immunoglobulin and com-plement), and defects in this mechanism could be an important factor in the evolution of circulating immune complex disease. Macrophages possess bac-tericidal and cytotoxic activity; are involved in host resistance to infection and tumour growth; and act as secretory cells capable of synthesizing and releasing hydrolytic enzymes as well as certain complement components and prostaglan-dins, all of which participate in inflammatory reactions (see Chapter 2).

Hypersensitivity reactions to antigens

A simple classification has been devised by Coombs and Gell (1975).

TYPE I REACTIONS

Type I reactions are those in which an antigen reacts with sensitized mast cells and basophils passively coated with cytophilic antibody usually of IgE type, and triggers the release of stored vasoactive amines from these cells (e.g. histamine, slow reactive substance A, and other pharmacological mediators). Although known to be associated with allergic diseases of the respiratory tract and skin as well as anaphylaxis, such reactions are now also regarded as being of importance in initiating the increased vascular permeability (including that of glomerular capillaries) which leads to the deposition of immune complexes and vascular damage in the rabbit model of acute complex disease following injection of bovine serum albumin. Although not proven, such mechanisms could be of importance in the pathogenesis of certain syndromes in man, in which immune complex deposition in vessels is now regarded as a basic lesion; for example, serum sickness, various forms of immune-complex nephritis, vasculitis and arthritis following meningococcal and gonococcal infections, and autoimmune diseases of which systemic lupus erythematosus may be regarded as a prototype (Chapter 2).

TYPE II REACTIONS

Type II reactions are those in which an antibody is cytotoxic to a cell or membrane bearing a specific antigen. In such reactions, complement may act as an important co-factor necessary for completion of the tissue-damaging process on the surface of cell membranes (e.g. red cell lysis by anti-erythrocyte antibody). *In vitro* experiments indicate the possibility that mononuclear cells bearing immunoglobulin heavy chain (Fc) receptors on their surface (sometimes called K cells) also collaborate in attacking target cells coated with antibody; for example, the pathogenesis of cell damage in Hashimoto's disease may be brought about by this system.

Antibodies directed against cell membrane antigens may acquire a special significance in those rheumatic diseases (e.g. systemic lupus erythematosus and rheumatoid arthritis) suspected to be due to virus infection. For example, cells infected with virus carry virus-specific antigens which are expressed on the host cell membrane and, if coated with viral antibody (the virus being effective in stimulating specific antibody response), would be susceptible to complement or K cell lysis. Such mechanisms have not yet been proven to be of pathogenetic importance. Another example of type II cytotoxic reactions directed against lymphocytes and mediated by antibody (and complement) is represented by the action of lymphocytotoxins which occur in the sera of patients with SLE and other autoimmune diseases (Chapter 6). It has been suggested that these antibodies may play an important role in altering lymphocyte function.

An unusual activity of antibody on cell membranes which leads to alteration in cell function has been included in this general category of reactions by Coombs and Gell. The stimulatory effect of the antibody 'long-acting thyroid stimulator' on thyroid-hormone-secreting cells is an example; a similar antibody-dependent basis for increased lysosomal production by chondrocytes of cartilage fragments in culture has been suggested by Coombs, Dingle and Fell (see Chapter 7). The demonstration of an antibody directed against the motor end-plate of the neuro-muscular junction may be of importance in myasthenia gravis (Chapter 8).

TYPE III REACTIONS

Type III reactions almost certainly play an important part in a number of rheumatic diseases. In these reactions freely dispersed antigen and antibody molecules form complexes either in circulating blood or in tissues. The circulating complexes lodge in target organs (e.g. blood vessels and kidneys) by mechanisms which are not very clearly understood, and initiate tissue damage. Complement probably plays an important role. Following binding of the first component of complement to the complex, and the resulting activation of the complement cascade system, a number of products are generated which have inflammatory and tissue damaging properties. Some, for example, lead to the release of vasoactive amines, which lead in turn to inflammation, others are chemotactic for polymorphs which are therefore attracted in large numbers to the site of the complexes. Here the polymorphs encounter the complexes where complement products facilitate their phagocytosis and release of lysosomal enzymes by various mechanisms. In certain infections microbial antigens form complexes with their antibody: these complexes circulate in blood and deposit in tissues where they mediate injury. Examples are the arthritis and vasculitis seen in hepatitis B infection and meningococcal septicaemia. Type III reactions are also believed to underlie the protean manifestations of SLE and the inflammatory responses observed in the joint in rheumatoid arthritis.

TYPE IV REACTIONS

Type IV reactions are mediated by interaction of antigen with receptor sites on T lymphocytes leading to the development of delayed hypersensitivity reactions. Activation of lymphocytes in this manner is associated with the acquisition by the lymphocyte of certain effector functions mediated by cell-to-cell contact or by generation of lymphokines, which have a number of biological activities including increased vascular permeability, inhibition of macrophage migration associated with macrophage activation, and stimulation and recruitment of other lymphocytes so that the response is amplified (Dumonde and Maini, 1971). By virtue of control of the microvasculature and permeability as well as local cellular accumulation and activity, type IV reactions lead to tissue damage. The demonstration of T cells and lymphokines in the rheumatoid joint has led to the speculation that these reactions may be of importance here. The proximity of mononuclear cells to necrotic muscle fibres in polymyositis has raised the possibility of direct cytotoxicity, further supported by the finding of circulating lymphocytes which are sensitized to muscle antigens. Although their importance in the rheumatic diseases remains largely conjectural at this stage, type IV reactions are a subject of considerable current research. Since T cells co-operate in the stimulation of antibody synthesis their part in initiating type III reactions is self-evident.

Genetic control of immune response and complement metabolism

The possibility of a genetic predisposition to rheumatic diseases has been pursued for a number of years utilizing epidemiological methods together with family and twin studies. Hitherto the evidence has not been strong for rheumatoid arthritis, is considerably better for SLE, and is undoubted in the case of ankylosing spondylitis. The possibility that the genetic factor operates via immune mechanisms has received support from the observation that ankylosing spondylitis is associated with HL-A-27 tissue type, because this locus is situated close to that which operates immune responses. Although the HL-A locus is close to the immune response gene in mice, the possibility that ankylosing spondylitis can be explained on this basis remains conjectural, since it remains to be shown that this condition is immunologically mediated. The occurrence of arthritis, bearing some resemblance to rheumatoid disease, in children with genetically inherited agammaglobulinaemia has been cited as supporting evidence for the presence of a genetic factor in rheumatoid arthritis working through the immune response. The clinical evidence for genetic influence in SLE is supported by the SLE-like syndromes seen in patients with hereditary deficiencies of certain complement components (for a full discussion see Chapter 13).

Cellular mechanisms of autoimmunity

Animal experiments indicate that autoantibody production can arise as a result of various events which terminate a previously unresponsive state to autoantigens. The following examples are chosen to illustrate some of the cellular mechanisms postulated as a basis for the emergence of autoimmunity.

BYPASS OF T CELL TOLERANCE

Unresponsiveness to autoantigens circulating in low amounts may be analogous to experimentally induced tolerance to antigens deliberately administered in a low dose over a continuous period. In this situation T cells become unresponsive and fail to interact with B cells, which in turn do not respond to autoantigens by proliferation and maturation into antibody-synthesizing cells. This situation is represented diagrammatically in Fig. 1.1a in which the tolerant T lymphocyte (Ta) is unresponsive to autoantigen (A), and the 'resting' sensitized B cell (Ba) does not produce anti-A antibody.

Specific T cell tolerance may be bypassed by an extrinsic cross-reacting antigen which happens to share some antigenic similarity with an autoantigen and thereby stimulates the resting B cell (see Allison, 1973). A possible means by which this may happen is shown diagrammatically in Fig. 1.1b in which the extrinsic antigen F-A (sharing antigen A with the challenged recipient) sets in train an immune response against only the foreign (F) component. A specifically sensitized T cell (Tf) responds and co-operates with its B cell counterpart (Bf) resulting in the production of anti-F antibody. The unexpected result of the interaction of antigen F-A, however, is that the T lymphocytes belonging to the set Tf also provide the necessary co-operation ('helper effect') for the set of lymphocytes (Ba) sensitized to autoantigens to produce anti-A antibody. This type of bypass may explain autoimmunity seen during infections with organisms possessing antigens which cross-react with host cells; for example, streptococcal infections leading to the production of anti-heart antibody in rheumatic fever. The presence of active B cells with unresponsiveness of T cells to autoantigens has been documented in rheumatic fever and other conditions (reviewed by Weigle, 1973).

The ability of viruses to invade mammalian cells and express their own specific antigens on the host cell membrane together with host-specific antigens is well

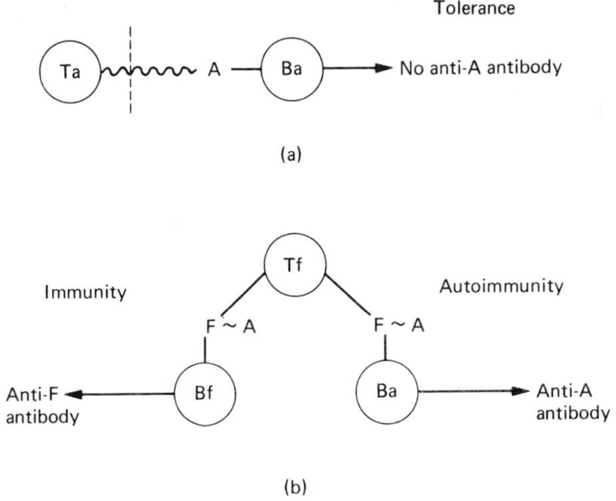

Fig. 1.1   (a) A diagrammatic representation of a 'tolerant' lymphocyte (Ta) bound to antigen; as a consequence of lack of T cell 'helper' function, no stimulation of Ba lymphocyte occurs. This mechanism appears to be a general phenomenon giving rise to 'tolerance' to autoantigens. (b) Mechanism of bypass of T cell tolerance by cross-reacting antigen F-A eliciting helper function for synthesis of anti-F and anti-A antibody.

recognized and could also result in the production of a combined unit of antigen corresponding to F-A described above, and similarly give rise to both virus-specific and autoantigen-specific antibodies. Thus the occurrence of antibodies which are cytotoxic for lymphocytes in the sera of New Zealand mice and patients with SLE and known virus infections could be explained on the basis of the expression of F-A-type antigen unit on infected lymphoid cells. Viruses, like streptococci, could also provide antigens which cross-react with host antigens (e.g. nucleic acids and proteins) by virtue of their own intrinsic molecular structure, or release autoantigens in large quantities from infected and damaged host tissues, so that low-dose tolerance is overcome. The ability of certain common virus infections in man (e.g. infectious mononucleosis and hepatitis B virus infections) to give rise to antibodies against smooth muscle and anti-nuclear antibodies is of possible relevance to this hypothesis.

Other mechanisms may also overcome T cell tolerance. For example, it has been suggested that immunological adjuvants (i.e. substances which increase specific immunological reactivity) can cause non-specific stimulation of T cells as well as stimulating the 'resting' B cells to form autoantibody. Experimental models of autoimmune diseases, such as thyroiditis, orchitis, allergic encephalomyelitis and arthritis, all require administration of the appropriate autoantigen in Freund's adjuvant (which consists of an emulsion of mineral oil and *Mycobacterium tuberculosis*). It seems that mycobacteria are powerful adjuvants and may act in this manner in leprosy. Autoantibodies also occur in association with other infections, e.g. lactic dehydrogenase virus in Aleutian mink disease, protozoa in malaria, and spirochaetes in syphilis, thus explaining the presence of anti-nuclear antibodies, rheumatoid factor and other autoantibodies described in these infectious diseases.

Johnson *et al.* (1975) have suggested that in certain circumstances T cell tolerance to autoantigens may be bypassed, and normally responsive (competent) B cells are directly stimulated, provided the antigen binding to its specific receptor is of high affinity. It has been hypothesized by these authors that this set of circumstances prevails in patients with rheumatoid arthritis by virtue of the presence in their serum of structurally altered IgG. A conformational alteration at or near the 'hinge' region of rheumatoid IgG has been demonstrated (by comparison with normal IgG) in physicochemical studies and by its localization in germinal centres of lymph nodes of mice following intraperitoneal injection. It is envisaged that the altered structure leads to binding of autologous IgG to Fc receptors on all B lymphocytes and a more efficient binding of antigenic determinants on the heavy chains which interact with the specifically sensitized subpopulation of B cells which are activated into cells which synthesize anti-globulin antibodies (rheumatoid factors), without T cell participation.

INTRINSIC ABNORMALITIES OF CELLULAR AND HUMORAL IMMUNOREGULATION

In the example cited above, autoimmunity results from environmental factors exerting their effects on a normally functioning immune system. Observations on the New Zealand (NZ) strains of mice led Talal (1970) to postulate the theory that a state of immunological imbalance leading to autoimmunity is expressed by defects of cellular and humoral immunity. In these animals, genetic influences are very evident and forceful evidence incriminating a viral aetiology for their autoimmune disease has been presented. Abnormalities of immunological reactivity (compared to controls) include: excessive antibody production to heterologous serum proteins and synthetic ribonucleic acids; difficulty in induction and maintenance of tolerance; impaired ability of NZ spleen cells to induce graft-versus-host reactions; impairment of lymphocyte responses to mitogens *in vitro* and impairment of ability to reject tumours. More direct evidence of abnormal immunological function of bone marrow and thymus cells has been produced. It is concluded by Talal that these experiments indicate a state of depressed cellular immunity and augmented antibody responses created by genetic and viral influences and leading to a predisposition to autoimmunity. Figure 1.2 illustrates the modified T and B cells in NZ mice responding to nuclear antigens by producing excessive anti-nuclear antibodies; the abnormal T cell functionally overcoming its unresponsive state and co-operating with B cells, and the latter being over-responsive to the stimulus. This simplified model does not attempt any explanation of the precise nature of the defects or examine the possibility that the nuclear antigens may be of viral origin and themselves immunogenic.

The autoimmune disease in NZ mice resembles SLE in several respects, in particular in the occurrence of anti-nuclear antibodies which are suspected to be deposited in the form of immune complexes in kidneys.

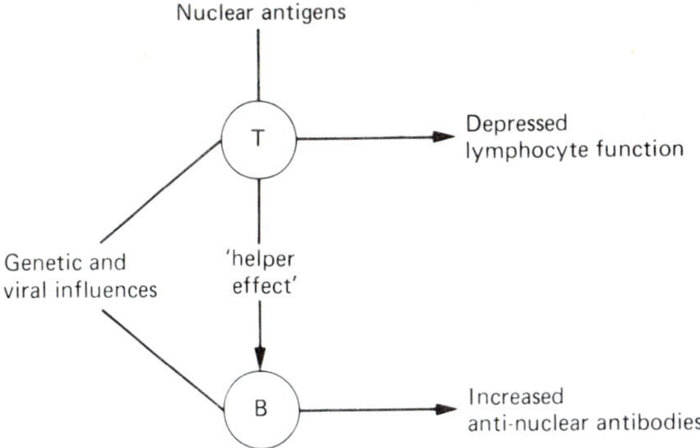

Fig. 1.2 Autoimmunity: abnormalities of T and B cells.

LOSS OF SUPPRESSOR T CELL FUNCTION

It will be appreciated that loss or bypass of T cell tolerance to autoantigens might
easily occur for a number of reasons; as a consequence the mechanism of tolerance
to autoantigens is not entirely secure. Several workers, including Allison and his
colleagues (1971), have hypothesized that T cells may provide an additional
means of controlling B cells in such circumstances by suppressing B-cell-
dependent synthesis of autoantibody. Loss of suppressor T cell function might
be expected to contribute to autoimmunity (Fig. 1.3) and evidence is currently

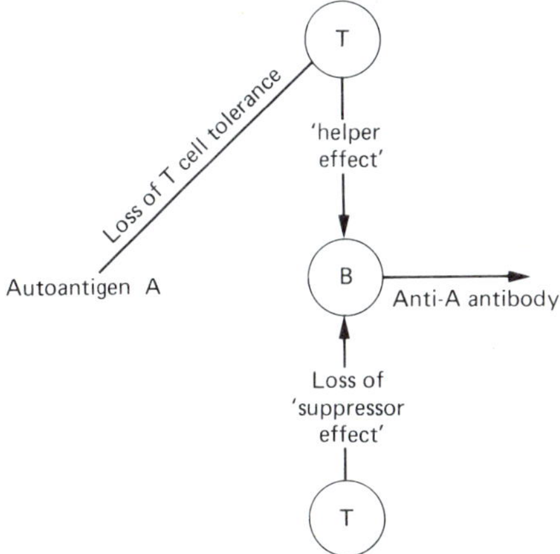

Fig. 1.3 Autoimmunity: loss of suppressor T cell function.

accumulating that such activity can indeed be demonstrated to reside in a T cell
population. For example, following early thymectomy which depletes T cells,

leghorn chickens develop a more severe form of autoimmune thyroiditis than occurs spontaneously (Welch *et al.*, 1973), and NZ mice manifest autoimmunity earlier (Talal, 1970). Transfer of lymphoid cells from old NZ black-strain mice suffering from autoimmune haemolytic anaemia (and lacking the putative suppressor T cells) into syngeneic young mice is followed by the development of a positive Coombs' test which is, however, short-lived; pretreatment of the young mice with anti-lymphocyte serum leads to a long-lived Coombs' test (evidence reviewed by Allison, 1973). It has been suggested that the results of these and other experiments support the presence of suppressor T cells.

The extent to which this type of defect might exist in rheumatic diseases is unknown, as is its possible relationship to other types of abnormalities which could lead to autoimmunity. The relevance of the depression of T cell numbers and lymphocyte-mediated responses documented in SLE (Chapter 6) to these experiments is speculative at present.

References

ADA, G. L. and PARISH, C. R. (1968). *Proc. nat. Acad. Sci. (Wash.)*, **61**, 556.

ALLISON, A. C. (1971). *Lancet*, **2**, 1401.

ALLISON, A. C. (1973). *Ann. rheum. Dis.*, **32**, 283.

ALLISON, A. C., DENMAN, A. M. and BARNES, R. D. (1971). *Lancet*, **2**, 135.

BURNET, F. M. (1959). *The Clonal Selection Theory of Acquired Immunity*. Cambridge University Press, Cambridge.

COOMBS, R. R. A. and GELL, P. G. H. (1975). In *Clinical Aspects of Immunology*, 3rd edn., p. 761. Ed. P. G. H. Gell, R. R. A. Coombs and P. J. Lachmann. Blackwell Scientific Publications, Oxford.

DRESSER, D. W. and MITCHISON, N. A. (1968). *Adv. Immunol.*, **8**, 129.

DUKOR, P., SCHUMANN, G., GISLER, R. H., DIERICH, M., KONIG, W., HADDING, U. and BITTER-SUERMANN, D. (1974). *J. exp. Med.*, **139**, 337.

DUMONDE, D. C. and MAINI, R. N. (1971). *Clin. Allergy*, **1**, 123.

FELDMANN, M. and NOSSAL, G. J. V. (1972). *Transplant Rev.*, **13**, 3.

JOHNSON, P. W., WATKINS, J. and HOLBOROW, E. J. (1975). *Lancet*, **1**, 611.

ROITT, I. M., GREAVES, M. F., TORRIGIANI, G., BROSTOFF, J. and PLAYFAIR, J. H. (1969). *Lancet*, **2**, 367.

TALAL, N. (1970). *Arthr. and Rheum.*, **13**, 887.

UNANUE, E. R. (1972). *Adv. Immunol.*, **15**, 95.

WEIGLE, W. O. (1973). *Adv. Immunol.*, **16**, 61.

WELCH, P., ROSE, N. R. and KITE, J. H. (1973). *J. Immunol.*, **110**, 575.

2

Mechanisms of Tissue Injury

Pathophysiology of tissue damage

In this chapter, the term 'tissue damage' is defined in clinicopathological terms, and is used to describe alterations in the normal biology of vascular, cellular and matrix components of tissues. The extent and the manner in which immune mechanisms may lead to such changes will be considered, but it is first necessary to examine the basic processes which are observed in the affected tissues.

VASCULAR DAMAGE

Damage to blood vessels can lead to:
1. transient and reversible dilatation of vessels and increased capillary permeability allowing escape of plasma proteins and blood cells (i.e. signs of acute inflammation);
2. vasculitis (i.e. morphological alteration in structure of blood vessels) of varying degrees and types affecting different sizes of arteries and veins as well as capillaries. Such changes include deposition of macromolecular space-occupying immune complexes; infiltration of the vessel wall with polymorphs and mononuclear cells; fibrinoid necrosis; deposition of fibrin; degeneration of collagen and elastin; fibrogenesis; intimal hyperplasia; vascular thrombotic occlusion; vascular rupture and avascular necrosis of tissues.

Clinical effects of vasculitis result from (a) widespread inflammation of blood vessels, and (b) ischaemia consequent upon vascular occlusion. These effects include skin lesions (maculopapular rashes, livedo reticularis, purpura, infarcts, ulcers); peripheral gangrene; and visceral lesions (infarction or necrosis, or more subtle metabolic change, leading to dysfunction of the heart, gastrointestinal tract, kidneys, brain, spinal cord and peripheral nerves).

CELLULAR DAMAGE

Cells may undergo necrosis or suffer damage owing not only to interference with blood supply, but also as a result of direct cytotoxic immune mechanisms (see Chapter 1, section on 'Hypersensitivity reactions'). Changes of repair and regeneration, fibrosis, lymphocyte, plasma cell and macrophage infiltration are seen in addition to the actual cellular damage itself, and the over-all picture is the result of a combination of processes.

MATRIX DAMAGE

The matrix of soft tissues composed of collagen, elastin and other materials (e.g. basement membrane) may degenerate or dissolve mainly as a result of enzymatic degradation leading to loss of normal framework and architecture. In the case of cartilage, matrix is composed of a fibrous component consisting of collagen and an amorphous component consisting partly of proteoglycan; both components may be enzymatically degraded. In the case of bone, erosion and collapse occur due to a combination of factors; e.g. vascular ischaemia, enzymatic degradation, increased osteoclastic activity and mechanical forces.

The immunological mechanisms which are believed to play an important part in the tissue-damaging processes of rheumatic disease mainly involve immune complexes and immune cells. The two processes are examined in detail separately, below.

Immune complexes and tissue damage

FORMATION AND DEPOSITION OF IMMUNE COMPLEXES

The concept that union of freely dispersed antigen and antibody (an immune complex) can mediate inflammatory reactions and lead to tissue damage is based on classical experimental observations. In the Arthus phenomenon (described in 1903), injection of antigen into the skin of previously immunized animals, whose blood was rich in precipitating antibody, led within a few hours to the appearance of an inflammatory reaction which could be severe enough to cause tissue necrosis. The administration to patients of antisera, raised in animals, against infective agents such as diphtheria and tetanus was also observed during the early part of the century to sometimes lead to 'serum sickness', a self-limiting disease characterized by fever, skin rashes, lymphadenopathy, polyarthritis and proteinuria. Models of this type of disease were described in animals following the administration of protein antigens, and a counterpart of 'acute' serum sickness in the rabbit was recognized following a single large dose of bovine serum albumin as was the 'chronic' development of glomerulonephritis following repeated injections of antigen in smaller doses, a subject fully reviewed by Weigle (1961), Unanue and Dixon (1967), and Cochrane and Koffler (1973).

Immune complexes can form at two main sites in the body, thus determining the subsequent pattern of organ or tissue involvement:

1. The complexes may be formed directly following introduction of antigen (as in the Arthus reaction) which remains localized in the tissues and combines with antibody which has been extravasated from the circulation. The reverse

sequence is equally effective, as demonstrated by the injection of antibody into the tissue in the presence of abundant circulating antigen, a model which may have important clinical implications in situations in which antibody synthesis may occur in diseased tissues (e.g. synovial membrane in rheumatoid arthritis).

2. The complexes may form in the blood stream and subsequently localize in tissues. Such a pattern is seen in the acute and chronic models of serum sickness. The presence of complexes in the blood stream provides an explanation for the multisystem features, as well as the localization of disease in blood vessels, endocardium and glomerular basement membrane.

The persistence of immune complexes for a sufficient period to permit localization in tissues depends upon a balance between their rates of generation and clearance by the reticuloendothelial system. The circumstances leading to persistence are not fully understood but include: excessive production, which presupposes a constant supply of antigen and antibody; intrinsic physical and biological properties of complexes retarding clearance by the reticuloendothelial system; and impaired function of the reticuloendothelial system itself. There is some evidence to support all three possibilities, but their precise individual roles remain uncertain.

The factors which lead to localization of circulating complexes in certain organs and tissues also remain largely unknown. It has been suggested that pressure and hydrodynamic forces may be important and account for deposition in glomerular walls and the bifurcation of vessels. Increased vascular permeability may be brought about by the action of histamine released from platelets, which in turn may be mediated by an intermediary factor (platelet-aggregating factor) released by basophils passively coated with IgE antibody reacting with antigen (Benveniste *et al.*, 1972). Complement-derived factors may also play an important part in generating vasoactive amines (see below). In the rabbit model of acute serum sickness early treatment with antagonists of vasoactive amines inhibits the emergence of arteritis and glomerulonephritis (Kniker and Cochrane, 1968). Glomerulonephritis in the chronic model was also largely prevented by such antagonists (Kniker, 1968) and established nephritis improved (Kniker, 1970). Although it seems likely that in immune complex diseases in man increased vascular permeability might occur as a prerequisite to deposition of complexes, the nature of the putative mediators and mechanisms involved is obscure.

PATHOGENESIS OF TISSUE INJURY

Not all immune complexes possess serious tissue-damaging potential. They are probably generated whenever any antigenic material finds access to the circulating blood in the presence of antibody, as is likely to occur, for example, during infections. In this situation elimination of complexes is achieved without any serious consequences, perhaps before any significant tissue fixation can occur. Kunkel has pointed out that in certain patients with a benign form of purpura (without any systemic disease) the serum contains very large quantities of immune complexes detectable as an intermediate-sized complex on analytical ultracentrifugation (Capra *et al.*, 1971). The complexes are not otherwise of any very serious consequence (see page 27).

In experimental animals, the circulating complexes that appear to be most toxic are soluble and formed in some antigen excess (Dixon *et al.*, 1961; Cochrane and Hawkins, 1968; Wilson and Dixon, 1971). The relative numbers, valency and size of molecules of antigen and antibody (itself bivalent if IgG or IgA, and pentavalent if IgM) determine whether the resulting immune complex will form a 'lattice' structure (which will precipitate) or remain in solution. In general, precipitates form at equivalence and antibody excess whereas soluble complexes are formed in antigen excess, though occasionally in antibody excess. The large precipitate is biologically inert or rapidly phagocytosed by cells of the reticulo-endothelial system and cleared from the circulation. The soluble complexes which are most toxic are nevertheless relatively large (sedimenting in the $>19S$ position on ultracentrifugation) and are formed in moderate antigen excess (e.g. $\times 20$ for albumin–anti-albumin), whereas the small soluble complexes form in great antigen excess (corresponding to molecules sedimenting at $<11S$ in the ultracentrifuge) seem to be less toxic. It is of some interest that the potentially most toxic complexes are also the most rapidly cleared, a reflection of an appropriately efficient defence mechanism. Mannik *et al.* (1974) have suggested that 'size' of complexes is not important in itself, but that the large complexes are usually more readily cleared because of their increased affinity for macrophage receptors. There is also the intriguing possibility that the larger, damaging, tissue-fixed complexes may be converted into small non-toxic complexes by the administration of excess amounts of antigen (Wilson and Dixon, 1971). The 'quality' of the antibody appears also to be of importance in its potential toxicity; non-precipitating antibodies correlated with severity of renal lesions in one study (Pincus *et al.*, 1968).

Once fixed in tissues (or blood vessels), immune complexes appear to require the participation of complement and phagocytic cells to initiate tissue damage, at least in experimental models. Thus, the Arthus reaction can be inhibited by the depletion of circulating polymorphs with nitrogen mustard. The arteritis observed in the rabbit model of acute serum sickness can also be inhibited by the depletion of polymorphs and the removal of complement from plasma by the administration of cobra venom. However, complement and polymorph depletion does not arrest the development of glomerular injury in acute serum sickness, indicating that other, as yet undefined, processes are involved (for references see Cochrane and Koffler, 1973).

The mechanisms of tissue injury involving complement and phagocytic cells are examined below.

ROLE OF COMPLEMENT

The complement system in blood consists of at least nine proteins and three enzyme-inhibitor systems. These proteins normally exist in an inactive form, but can be activated in a variety of ways, including the combination of immune complexes with the first component of complement, C1. This leads to a sequential involvement of C4, 2, 3, 5, 6, 7, 8 and 9 components and results in the generation of a number of products which are relevant to tissue injury (see page 41. For a review see Alper, 1974).

1. C3a and C5a derived by cleavage of C3 and C5 respectively possess 'anaphylotoxin' activity by virtue of their ability to release vasoactive amines from mast cells. Increased vascular permeability can also result from the direct action of a kinin-like activity derived from C2 complement component. Increased vascular permeability not only gives rise to signs of acute inflammation, but is also a critical factor in the localization of circulating immune complexes.

2. The assembly of C5–9 components of complement bound to the cell membranes leads to cytolysis.

3. The generation in the fluid phase of C5a and the trimolecular complex C567 from inactive complement precursors provide molecules which possess strong chemotactic activity. This activity is responsible for the attraction of large numbers of polymorphs to the site of the complex.

4. The action of the enzymatic activities generated from the 'classical' and the 'alternate' pathways on complement component C3 gives rise to the molecule C3b which, attached to the immune complex, acts as an 'opsonin' and encourages immune adherence to phagocytes. Phagocytosis of immune complexes is associated with the release of acid hydrolases which enzymatically digest constituents of connective tissue (see below).

ROLE OF POLYMORPHONUCLEAR NEUTROPHILS AND MACROPHAGES

The polymorph is the predominant cell in the Arthus type reaction. Phagocytosis of immune complexes by polymorphs *in vitro* occurs without loss of cell viability and is accompanied by degranulation of lysosomes and release of hydrolytic enzymes which can break down connective tissue matrix (Henson, 1971; Weissmann, 1972). Polymorphs also adhere to immune complexes on intact surfaces such as vascular basement membranes and selectively release lysosomal enzymes by a process which is termed 'reverse endocytosis'. This follows binding of the Fc part of the immunoglobulin in the complex to a surface receptor on the cell, and can occur in the absence of complement. However, some complexes and particles can only be efficiently phagocytosed provided they are opsonized by the C3b product of complement activation. In addition, a molecule similar to C5a may act as a lysosomal-releasing factor.

The monocyte (or macrophage) is not usually encountered in the arteritic and glomerular lesions in the models of immune complex diseases described previously. In the diseased synovium of rheumatoid arthritis, however, local antibody synthesis and immune complex formation do occur, and in this situation the phagocytic cells of the lining layer and mononuclear phagocytes in the tissues may be important sources of hydrolytic enzymes (Allison *et al.*, 1975). It has been shown *in vitro* that macrophages, like polymorphs, secrete lysosomal enzymes when exposed to preformed immune complexes. These include neutral proteases that can degrade connective tissue components, such as collagen.

Cell-mediated tissue injury

PATHOGENESIS

The functional activity of lymphocytes represents a delicate balance resulting from many different mechanisms. On the one hand, the concept of hypofunctional lymphocytes is central to the development of autoimmune responses and breakdown of tolerance, as is discussed further in Chapter 3. On the other hand, there is little doubt that some form of over-activity is implicated in the allergic tissue-damaging reactions mediated by lymphocytes.

The possibility that lymphocytes are directly involved in the pathogenesis of human connective tissue diseases and in experimentally induced autoimmune diseases is supported by several observations. For example:

1. A disease resembling rheumatoid arthritis in some respects occurs in children with immunodeficiency characterized by agammaglobulinaemia with preservation of lymphocyte function.

2. The histological appearance of synovial membrane in rheumatoid arthritis shows infiltration with lymphocytes and plasma cells, and the abundance of lymphocytes is related to the extent to which complement is lowered in synovial fluid; this, in turn, is related to severity of joint damage (Schur *et al.*, 1975).

3. The products of lymphocyte activation (i.e. lymphokines) have been demonstrated in the synovial fluid of patients with rheumatoid arthritis; rheumatoid synovial explant cultures synthesize lymphokines suggesting their continual production; and injection of lymphokine-like material into rabbit knee joints induces a chronic synovitis (Stastny *et al.*, 1975).

4. The close physical association of lymphocytes with areas of necrotic muscle tissue in polymyositis (see page 95) suggests an aggressor role for these cells, as does their presence in cartilage in cases of polychondritis (see page 101). The presence of lymphocytes in the erosive lesion of ankylosing spondylitis at the junction of bone and ligament may be a comparable phenomenon.

5. Lymphocyte depletion by thoracic duct drainage in patients with rheumatoid arthritis leads to remission of symptoms (Paulus *et al.*, 1973).

6. Introduction of antigen into the ankle joints of previously sensitized chickens produced a chronic synovitis in bursectomized (and hence agammaglobulinaemic) birds (Oates *et al.*, 1973).

7. Allergic encephalomyelitis, allergic thyroiditis and adjuvant arthritis can be induced in animals by transfer of lymphocytes from diseased animals.

It should not, however, be assumed from the examples quoted above that a single class of lymphocytes is responsible for mediating the disease process. Many different cell types, including several subpopulations of lymphocytes as well as macrophages and polymorphs, are likely to be involved. Certain cellular reactions seem also to require the direct participation of antibody and complement. Indeed, sites of allergic reactions may at one and the same time show evidence of cellular- (type IV) and antibody-mediated (type III) inflammation or tissue damage.

Different orders of specificity are involved in damage to tissues by cellular immune mechanisms. For example:

1. Specifically sensitized lymphocytes may damage tissues bearing appropriate antigen.

2. Specifically sensitized lymphocytes when activated produce mediators with specificity for certain types of cells or tissues; e.g. the effects of different lymphokines on macrophages, polymorphs or blood vessels.

3. Lymphocytes and macrophages may interact in a non-specific way, but liberate enzymes which have their own tissue-degrading specificity; e.g. the action of lysosomal hydrolases on cartilage, elastin and collagen.

In contrast, the consequences of other cellular reactions are entirely non-specific; for example, activated macrophages are cytotoxic for any micro-organism or tumour, and 'lymphotoxin' for any cell (see below). The importance of these mainly *in vitro* observations lies in providing a conceptual framework for the better understanding of *in vivo* events, but it has to be pointed out that their relevance to disease processes remains, as yet, largely conjectural.

MECHANISMS OF CELL-MEDIATED CYTOTOXICITY

The following general methods have been used to study cellular injury in culture: (1) assessment of cellular death (e.g. by measuring viability or release of radio-labelled chromium); (2) measurement of depression of cellular metabolism (e.g. protein synthesis); (3) inhibition of growth and reproduction of cells (e.g. clonal inhibition). The mechanisms of cellular injury are considered below, but for details the reader is referred to the excellent reviews by Cerottini and Brunner (1974) and Perlmann and Holm (1969).

(a) Specifically sensitized lymphocyte-mediated cytotoxicity

This reaction is mediated by specifically sensitized T cells reacting with appropriate antigens on the surface of target cells, as exemplified by allograft reactions.

(b) Activation of lymphocytes

Culture of any target cell in the presence of lymphocytes which have been activated by antigen or mitogens (e.g. tuberculin PPD or PHA) leads to target cell lysis, a reaction described as the 'innocent bystander' cytotoxicity.

(c) Lymphotoxin

The supernatants of antigen- or mitogen-activated lymphocytes generate a soluble factor which resembles other lymphokines, and is termed 'lymphotoxin' because of its cytotoxicity for any cells cultured with the material. It is postulated that lymphotoxin may be the effector molecule for (b), above.

(d) *Antibody-dependent mononuclear cell cytotoxicity*

In the presence of a very low amount of specific antibody coating a target cell, mononuclear cells mediate cytotoxicity. The mononuclear cells responsible have been separated and characterized as being non-phagocytic; and it is generally agreed that they do not possess surface immunoglobulin (i.e. they are not B cells) nor do they carry T cell receptors. They do, however, carry a receptor for the Fc part of the heavy chains of IgG and thus appear to constitute a distinct population of lymphocytes referred to as 'K' cells. The cytotoxic reaction does not require complement and apparently takes place by binding of the Fc receptor to the heavy chain of immunoglobulin already attached to the target cells. The reaction is inhibited by rheumatoid factors and immune complexes which compete for the reactive binding sites. It is worthy of note that B cells, monocytes (or macrophages) and polymorphs also carry Fc receptors on their membranes, and, under appropriate conditions, can also bind and damage antibody-coated target cells. Indeed, the possibility has been considered that the apparently distinct K cell population may be either a subclass of B cells or monocytes which have not adapted to a phagocytic function.

(e) *Macrophage and polymorphonuclear cell-mediated cytotoxicity*

Stimulation of lymphocytes by antigen and mitogens leads to the generation of mediators with a variety of biological activities, including factors which affect macrophage function. Macrophages activated by lymphocyte-derived mediators *in vitro* acquire an increased non-specific microbicidal activity, and it is believed that this activity is relevant to acquired resistance mediated by lymphocytes and macrophages to infection *in vivo* (Mackaness, 1971). The extent to which physical proximity between lymphocytes and macrophages is necessary for these reactions remains unclear.

Peritoneal macrophages from mice immunized with tumour cells were found to inhibit growth and showed cytotoxicity towards the same tumour *in vitro*. Normal macrophages incubated with hyperimmune lymphoid cells for 24 hours could also mediate cytotoxicity which was specific for the tumour cell used for immunization, the procedure of incubation leading to 'arming' of the macrophage (Evans and Alexander, 1970). Immune lymphocytes (believed to be T cells) incubated with the tumour cell (as antigen) for 24 hours produced a soluble factor in the supernatants of the cultures which was termed the 'specific macrophage arming factor' (SMAF). This soluble factor has the capacity of rendering normal macrophages specifically cytotoxic for the tumour cells *in vitro*, and in this respect differs from the non-specificity of the bactericidal activity of activated macrophages. However, it has been shown that once the armed macrophages have encountered their specific antigen on target cells, they become capable of exerting non-specific cytotoxicity towards other tumour cells in culture.

The ability of antibody-coated (opsonized) tissue cells to attach to the Fc receptor of macrophages and polymorphs offers another mechanism whereby a cell is damaged. This interaction leads to release of tissue-damaging lysosomal enzymes, whether or not phagocytosis occurs.

ADDITIONAL FORMS OF CELL-MEDIATED TISSUE INJURY

Apart from their direct cytotoxic potential, lymphocytes and macrophages may contribute to tissue damage in other ways. For example, lymphokines derived from lymphocytes, and antibody (a B lymphocyte product) as part of immune complexes, interact with polymorphs and macrophages and lead to synthesis and release of lysosomal enzymes which are capable of degrading connective tissue components and mediating other effects discussed in a previous part of this chapter. Recent evidence has implicated macrophages in the synthesis of prostaglandin, a potent inflammatory mediator, and other types of lymphocyte–macrophage interaction have been suggested (Morley *et al.*, 1975). Macrophages under certain situations promote fibrogenesis (Allison *et al.*, 1975). When viewed together, it may be appreciated that cellular processes are of great importance in the pathogenesis of connective tissue disease lesions.

References

ALLISON, A. C., CARDELLA, C. and DAVIES, P. (1975). *Rheumatology*, **6**, 251.

ALPER, C. A. (1974). In *The Structure and Function of Proteins*, p. 195. Ed. A. C. Allison. Academic Press, New York and London.

BENVENISTE, J., HENSON, P. M. and COCHRANE, C. G. (1972). *J. exp. Med.*, **136**, 1356.

CAPRA, J. D., WINCHESTER, R. J. and KUNKEL, H. G. (1971). *Medicine (Baltimore)*, **50**, 125.

CEROTTINI, J. C. and BRUNNER, T. (1974). *Adv. Immunol.*, **18**, 67.

COCHRANE, C. G. and HAWKINS, D. (1968). *J. exp. Med.*, **127**, 137.

COCHRANE, C. G. and KOFFLER, D. (1973). *Adv. Immunol.*, **16**, 186.

DIXON, F. J., FELDMAN, J. D. and VAZQUEZ, J. J. (1961). *J. exp. Med.*, **113**, 899.

EVANS, R. and ALEXANDER, P. (1970). *Nature (Lond.)*, **228**, 620.

HENSON, P. M. (1971). *J. exp. Med.*, **134**, 114 (s).

KNIKER, W. T. (1968). *Fed. Proc.*, **27** (2), 409.

KNIKER, W. T. (1970). *Fed. Proc.*, **29** (2), 287.

KNIKER, W. T. and COCHRANE, C. G. (1968). *J. exp. Med.* **127**, 119.

MACKANESS, G. B. (1971). In *Progress in Immunology*, Vol. I, p. 413. Ed. B. Amos. Academic Press, New York and London.

MANNIK, M., HAAKENSTAD, A. O. and AREND, W. P. (1974). In *Progress in Immunology*, Vol. II, 5, p. 57. Ed. L. Brent and J. Holborow. North Holland Publishing Co., Amsterdam.

MORLEY, J., BRAY, M. A., GORDON, D. and PAUL, W. (1975). In *The Immunological Basis of Connective Tissue Diseases*, p. 115. Ed. L. G. Silvestri. North Holland Publishing Co., Amsterdam.

OATES, C. M., MAINI, R. N., PAYNE, L. N. and DUMONDE, D. C. (1973). In *Microenvironmental Aspects of Immunity*, p. 611. Ed. B. D. Jankovic and K. Isakovic. Plenum, New York and London.

PAULUS, H. E., MACHLEDER, H., BANGERT, R., STRATTON, J., GOLDBERG, L., WHITEHOUSE, M. W., YU, D. and PEARSON, C. M. (1973). *Clin. Immunol. Immunopathol.*, **1**, 173.

PERLMANN, P. and HOLM, G. (1969). *Adv. Immunol.*, **11**, 117.

PINCUS, T., HABERKERN, R. and CHRISTIAN, C. L. (1968). *J. exp. Med.*, **127**, 819.

SCHUR, P. H., BRITTON, M. C., FRANCO, A. E., CORSON, J. M., SOSMAN, J. L. and RUDDY, S. (1975). *Rheumatology*, **6**, 34.

STASTNY, P., ROSENTHAL, M., ANDREIS, M., COOKE, D. and ZIFF, M. (1975). *Ann. N.Y. Acad. Sci.*, **256**, 117.

UNANUE, E. R. and DIXON, F. J. (1967). *Adv. Immunol.*, **6**, 1.

WEIGLE, W. O. (1961). *Adv. Immunol.*, **1**, 283.

WEISSMANN, G. (1972). *New Engl. J. Med.*, **286**, 141.

WILSON, C. B. and DIXON, F. J. (1971). *J. exp. Med.*, **134**, 7 (s).

3

Immune Reactions to Autoantigens

Autoantibodies

The detection of antibodies directed against autoantigens in patients with diseases such as Hashimoto's thyroiditis, rheumatoid arthritis and systemic lupus erythematosus was largely responsible for the emergence of the concept that autoimmune processes may be of pathogenetic importance. Experience has shown, however, that autoantibodies are not unique to these diseases, and occur even in apparently healthy individuals and are therefore not necessarily of pathogenetic importance. Nevertheless, it seems that autoantibodies in disease and health might differ from each other in quantity, quality and possibly reactivity against certain specific antigens. If they possess pathogenetic potential at all, it is likely that it would be expressed by type II or type III reactions (discussed in this section). The so-called 'organ-specific' antibodies (e.g. thyroid or red cell antibodies) tend to be implicated in type II reactions, whereas 'non-organ-specific' antibodies mediate damage by forming immune complexes which are a characteristic feature of the diseases discussed in this book.

The autoantibodies that will be discussed in this chapter fall into the following main classes, defined on the basis of antigen specificity:

1. antibodies directed against antigenic determinants on immunoglobulin molecules (anti-globulin antibodies);

2. antibodies directed against antigenic constituents in the nucleus and cytoplasm;

3. antibodies to cartilage and connective tissue components, e.g. chondrocytes, proteoglycans and collagen.

Rheumatoid factors

NATURE AND OCCURRENCE

A large number of antibodies are described with specificity for antigenic sites on the immunoglobulin molecule, collectively termed 'anti-globulin factors'. Among these are rheumatoid factors, which are antibodies directed against antigenic sites on heavy chain determinants. These determinants have been located in the Fc portion as obtained by papain treatment of immunoglobulin. The part of the heavy chain obtained following this treatment is shown in Fig. 3.1; it comprises a sequence of amino acids termed the second (C_H2) and third (C_H3)

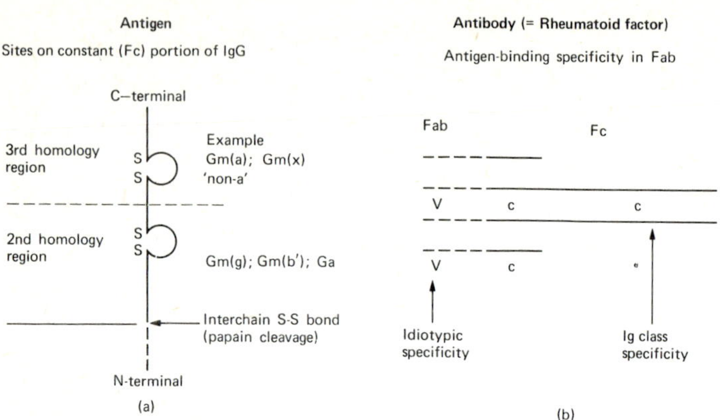

Fig. 3.1   Rheumatoid factors are antibodies directed against antigenic sites on constant portion of the heavy chain of IgG (**a**). Examples of antigenic sites are shown above. The rheumatoid factor (**b**) itself may belong to any of the described Ig classes, and the class specificity (e.g. IgG, IgM) will be determined by the heavy chain. Idiotypic specificity of rheumatoid factor is determined by raising antibodies to the variable portion of the rheumatoid factor itself.

homology regions of the constant part of the heavy chain, both regions possessing 'antigenic' sites for rheumatoid factor (Natvig *et al.*, 1972). Some of these antigenic sites are present only in certain groups of individuals and are under the control of alleles which are inherited according to classical Mendelian genetics and include the so-called Gm markers, whilst others are found in all sera but may be restricted to subclasses of IgG. These antigens include Gm (a), 'non-a' and Gm (x), which are present in the third homology region, and Gm (g) and Gm (b') and Ga which are present in the second homology region.

Rheumatoid factors in patients with rheumatoid arthritis are directed against antigenic sites present on autologous IgG (common specificities being Gm (a), 'non-a', and Ga) (Natvig *et al.*, 1971). Rheumatoid factors with specificities for non-autologous human IgG as well as antigenic sites present on immunoglobulins from other species (hetero-specific) also occur, and in individual patients rheumatoid factors of all these specificities have been described. Although rheumatoid factor combinations with immunoglobulins in the aggregated or denatured form are readily detectable by agglutination or precipitation reactions *in vitro*, rheumatoid factors also combine with IgG in its 'native' form but do not lead to agglutination or precipitation. The difference in reactivity appears to lie in the increased affinity of aggregated IgG for rheumatoid factor, possibly as a result of its polyvalent nature so that an appropriate lattice formation results in the observed physicochemical reactions.

In patients with rheumatoid arthritis, rheumatoid factors frequently combine with autologous IgG to form immune complexes in the blood and synovial tissue and fluid. IgM rheumatoid factor in serum circulates as large macromolecular (22S) complexes with IgG (Kunkel and Tan, 1964); in addition, IgG rheumatoid factor circulates as intermediate-sized (9–17S) complex (Capra *et al.*, 1971) and is a main component of synovial fluid complexes (Winchester *et al.*, 1970). Synovial tissue eluates in patients with rheumatoid arthritis were shown in a study by Natvig and others (1971) to frequently contain rheumatoid factor activity directed against autologous IgG which was only revealed by acid dissociation or pepsin digestion ('hidden rheumatoid factor'). Immunofluorescent studies on rheumatoid synovium also suggest that rheumatoid factor synthesized by plasma cells *in vivo* is 'blocked' by IgG–anti-IgG complex formation (Natvig *et al.*, 1975).

HETEROGENEITY

Rheumatoid factors are not only heterogeneous in respect of their specificity for different antigenic sites on IgG. Rheumatoid factor was long regarded as belonging exclusively to the IgM class of immunoglobulins, but more recently IgG, IgD and IgA rheumatoid factors have been demonstrated. Within each class rheumatoid factor may be homogeneous with respect to its electrophoretic mobility (monoclonal) or non-homogeneous (polyclonal). The affinity of rheumatoid factor for its antigen (immunoglobulin) is variable, presumably depending on whether the antibody forms a 'good fit' or a 'poor fit'. Other variables include valency (5 for IgM, 2 for IgG and IgA), and optimal temperature conditions under which antigen–antibody combination occurs (e.g. 4°C for IgG).

Rheumatoid factors with the same antibody-combining specificity for their antigens may nevertheless show subtle differences in the amino acid sequence structure of the variable part of their own immunoglobulin (marked 'V' in Fig. 3.1). This characteristic of the immunoglobulin is termed 'idiotypic specificity', and may be detected by raising specific antibodies in suitable animals.

Following combination with its antigen, rheumatoid factor has been shown to bind complement. For these studies it has been necessary to reduce and alkylate the immunoglobulin used as antigen to ensure that the complement binding was mediated only by the rheumatoid factor molecule. Both IgM and IgG rheumatoid factor have been shown to possess this capacity, but the variables include temperature conditions under which optimum fixation occurs, as well as the molarity of the respective reactants. It has also been shown that rheumatoid factors fix complement when derived from patients with rheumatoid arthritis but not from healthy individuals (Bianco *et al.*, 1974).

Since the heterogeneity of rheumatoid factors influences their biological activity, it may be expected that their diagnostic and pathogenetic importance will reflect such variation. However, the variety of tests for rheumatoid factors used in clinical practice at present usually detect IgM rheumatoid factor. The reactants used (e.g. rabbit amboceptor on sheep erythrocytes or latex coated with human immunoglobulin G or anti-D antibody coating human Rh-positive cells) could also favour detection of certain antigenic determinants or class of antibody, as would the temperature conditions. The procedures themselves are variable to an extent that incorporation of standard rheumatoid factors in every test is necessary, but these are not widely used in practice. A further complication arises from the fact that a serum factor (probably C1q component of complement) reacts with IgG, especially in latex agglutination tests, giving a false positive reaction. Heating the serum for 30 minutes at 56°C should inactivate C1q, however, and is a useful routine precaution.

IgM AND IgG RHEUMATOID FACTORS

Most of the population surveys that have been performed were carried out with tests which detect a group of IgM rheumatoid factors. Of the tests that are extensively used, it has been shown that the Rose–Waaler test employing sentized sheep cells shows the greatest diagnostic specificity for rheumatoid arthritis but is only present in 60–70 per cent of patients. However, patients with a number of other diseases, as well as healthy individuals in the older age group, also possess rheumatoid factors (Bartfield, 1969) (also see Chapter 5).

Rheumatoid factors of the IgG class occur in health and disease, although levels in rheumatoid arthritis are higher (Panush *et al.*, 1971). This class of factor, however, is also found to be elevated in the so-called sero-negative patients with rheumatoid disease (usually Rose–Waaler or latex negative and therefore lacking IgM rheumatoid factor) (Howell *et al.*, 1972). Such disease categories include a polyarthritis resembling sero-positive rheumatoid arthritis in adults but lacking nodules, most forms of juvenile chronic polyarthritis, ankylosing spondylitis, psoriatic arthritis, enteropathic arthritis and Reiter's disease.

The methods employed for detecting IgG rheumatoid factors rely on the use of appropriate immunoabsorbents which bind IgG rheumatoid factors; the latter are subsequently separated from the immunoabsorbent by acid dissociation, and assayed against anti-IgG antibody by diffusion in agar. Various immunoabsorbents have been used, including Sepharose linked to IgG by cyanogen bromide and bis diazotized benzidine treated horse IgG.

CLINICAL SIGNIFICANCE

IgM rheumatoid factors detected by agglutination tests, apart from their diagnostic value, have been shown to correlate with: nodules; worse over-all prognosis; severe bone destruction in rheumatoid joints; multi-system involvement; and vasculitis.

Rheumatoid factors of IgG class complexed with IgG have been found in serum, synovial fluid and synovial membranes of patients with rheumatoid arthritis (Chapter 5). In synovial fluids, an inverse correlation between the amount of complexed IgG and total haemolytic complement activity was found by Winchester and his colleagues (1969, 1970). The complexes were of the type that bound with C1q component of complement and their capacity to activate complement was demonstrated by anticomplementary activity. In contrast to this finding it is noted that IgG complexes in serum are not associated with complement activation to the same degree, probably because they do not possess the physical configuration which allows efficient binding to C1q. 'Soluble' IgG complexes in synovial fluid become 'insoluble' when they interact with IgM rheumatoid factor; such insoluble complexes, especially in the presence of C3b fragment of activated C3 which facilitates 'immune adherence' to phagocytic cells, are phagocytosed and contribute to lysosomal enzyme release. The finding of IgG, IgM and C3 within phagocytic cells in synovial fluid and membrane lends support to this sequence of events.

However, the concept of a pathogenetic role for rheumatoid factors remains controversial, since these may occur in the serum of individuals without any arthritis or demonstrable disease, and furthermore it was found impossible to induce arthritis by infusion of IgM rheumatoid factor into volunteer healthy recipients (Harris and Vaughan, 1961). It has been suggested that IgM rheumatoid factor interaction with potentially tissue-damaging complexes should lead to a more efficient clearance by the reticuloendothelial system. A more convincing protective role for rheumatoid factor has been suggested on the basis of its property of virus neutralization *in vitro* (Notkins, 1971).

Complexes containing IgG rheumatoid factor of intermediate size (9–17S) have been regularly demonstrated in patients with the syndrome of hyperglobulinaemic purpura (Capra *et al.*, 1971). The intermediate size complexes arise from interactions of IgG rheumatoid factor (the 'antibody') with other IgG molecules (the 'antigen') in the serum, and appear to induce the purpuric lesions by poorly understood mechanisms. Similar complexes occur in patients with rheumatoid arthritis and this type of complex associated with IgM rheumatoid factor may lead to hyperviscosity of serum in certain patients with rheumatoid arthritis and account for symptoms of dyspnoea, weakness and a tendency to bleeding (Jasin *et al.*, 1970). In the syndrome of mixed IgG–IgM cryoglobulinaemia, purpura, arthralgias, lymphadenopathy, hepatosplenomegaly and glomerulonephritis occur; in this situation cryoglobulins are present in serum and possess rheumatoid factor activity and the complexes may fix complement (Meltzer and Franklin, 1966).

Other antiglobulin factors

Pepsin digestion of IgG molecules produces Fab$_2$ fragments which are immunogenic, and antibodies to these are termed 'pepsin agglutinators'. Complexes of pepsin agglutinator with its antigen have been found in rheumatoid synovial tissue and fluid, raising the possibility that they are of pathogenetic significance (Mellbye and Natvig, 1971; Munthe and Natvig, 1971). Indeed, some complement fixation was also noted to occur with such complexes *in vitro*. Injection of Fab fragments (papain-treated IgG) into the knee joints of rabbits led to an acute synovitis only if the injected rabbits also had homoreactants (specific antibody similar to pepsin agglutinators) in their serum (Rawson *et al.*, 1969). In this study, repeated injections induced a chronic synovitis with villous proliferation resembling rheumatoid arthritis. Lysosomal enzymes active at neutral pH of human origin have been demonstrated which degrade IgG into Fab-like fragments to which antibodies occur in rheumatoid sera (LoSpalluto *et al.*, 1970) and which, complexed with homoreactant antibody, appear to provide the stimulus for the production of rheumatoid factor by the synovium in rabbits (Fehr *et al.*, 1975). A direct correlation was shown between the level of homoreactant and rheumatoid factor titre by these workers. Thus this type of antibody may itself be of some importance in the production of inflammation, and lead to enhanced generation of rheumatoid factor.

Antibodies to chondrocytes

The possibility that cartilage damage in rheumatoid arthritis and osteoarthrosis may be partly mediated by immunological injury to chondrocytes was considered on the basis of certain *in vitro* observations by Dame Honor Fell and her colleagues. These experiments were performed on fragments of cartilage with a pig erythrocyte antiserum which cross-reacted with chondrocytes.

When the proteoglycan matrix of cartilage was first rendered permeable, the antiserum (in the presence of complement) induced increased metabolic activity or cell death of the chondrocytes, depending on the local concentration and degree of accessibility of the immunoglobulin (Fell and Barratt, 1973; Poole *et al.*, 1973). The matrix was rendered permeable by culturing joint capsule or marrow cells in the vicinity of the cartilage fragment and it was presumed that a factor generated by these soft tissues, possibly an enzyme derived from lysosomes, was responsible for matrix degradation. Such a mechanism was postulated in rheumatoid synovitis in which the hypertrophic synovium was thought to account for the loss of matrix, and the ubiquitous antichondrocyte antibody was considered to mediate chondrocyte necrosis, the latter being regarded as a significant lesion in rheumatoid arthritis by Kulka (1959). However, chondrocyte necrosis is not usually a feature of the cartilage in rheumatoid arthritis and it is uncertain whether such a mechanism is of any significance in the disease.

The possibility has also been considered that cartilage damage mediated by intermittent exposure to proteolytic enzymes and antichondrocyte antibodies eventually gives rise to changes in cartilage resembling osteoarthrosis (Millroy and Poole, 1974).

Antibodies to proteoglycans

The amorphous component of the matrix of cartilage is largely composed of macromolecules termed 'proteoglycans', which consist of a core of protein attached to polysaccharide side chains. Both antibody and lymphocyte-mediated responses to these molecules have been recognized and may be of pathogenetic importance in a rare disorder called relapsing polychondritis (Chapter 9).

Antibodies to collagen

Circulating antibodies to a soluble fraction of human collagen can be obtained by the immunization of experimental animals, and similar antibodies have been demonstrated in up to 40 per cent of rheumatoid arthritis sera (Steffen,1971). The finding of intracytoplasmic inclusion of collagen in synovial fluid exudate cells by these authors was taken as evidence suggesting that collagen linked to antibody may form complexes which are an additional class of autoantigen–antibody complexes present in the rheumatoid joint and involved in the inflammatory pathogenetic process. The demonstration of structural similarities between C1q component of complement and collagen noted by Calcott and Müller-Eberhard (1972) raises questions of the specificity of reactions attributed to collagen, and also gives rise to the interesting possibility that a soluble collagen similar to C1q might be synthesized by rheumatoid synovium and initiate complement activation.

Anti-nuclear antibodies

In 1948 the LE cell phenomenon was described as a diagnostic feature of systemic lupus erythematosus (SLE). Thereafter it became apparent that the LE cell phenomenon depended on the presence in the serum of antibody to nucleoprotein. Further investigations have shown that a number of cellular constituents may act as antigens and that antibodies to such antigens are found not only in patients with SLE, but also in a variety of other diseases, and even in apparently good health. Numerous techniques are employed for the demonstration of antibodies to a variety of nuclear antigens and their diagnostic specificity and possible role in the pathogenesis of disease has been extensively investigated in the past 20 years. The involvement of these antibodies in the pathogenesis of immune-complex-mediated lesions in SLE, especially in renal lesions, is considered in Chapter 6.

IMMUNOFLUORESCENT TESTS

Microtome sections of frozen rat liver are usually employed as the substrate for the detection of anti-nuclear antibodies by incubating them with the test serum. After a suitable period, fluorescein-conjugated antiglobulins are applied to demonstrate the site at which antibodies attached to the cell. Dilutions of the test serum are used to determine the titre of the serum which still gives a reaction with the tissue section, the higher titres being usually more clinically significant. Standard sera may be incorporated to express the results in units of activity. It is also possible to differentiate at least four staining patterns and, although these may be influenced by technical procedures, they are dependent to a certain extent on the nuclear antigen involved in the antibody reactions, and have a degree of diagnostic value (see Table 3.1). Thus, of the commonly observed patterns, the homogeneous (or diffuse) pattern of nuclear fluorescence correlates with positive LE cell tests. This type of reaction has been described in a large number of diseases; e.g. the majority of patients with SLE, in up to 25 per cent patients with rheumatoid arthritis (RA), in patients with chronic active hepatitis (20 per cent), frequently in Sjögren's syndrome, drug-induced SLE and myasthenia gravis. It is seen less commonly in leprosy, infectious mononucleosis and also in patients with extensive injuries or burns, pulmonary emboli, pregnancy and malignancy.

A 'speckled' pattern has been observed in sera of patients with scleroderma,

Table 3.1   Detection of antinuclear antibodies by immunofluorescent methods (tissue substrate—usually liver)

Pattern of nuclear staining	Antigens*	Comment*
Homogeneous	DNA-histone†	Commonest pattern; may mask other antibody patterns in same serum
Peripheral	DS-DNA	Rare; sera with antibodies to DS-DNA frequently do not show this reaction
Speckled	ENA	At least 2 antigens involved: trypsin and ribonuclease sensitive (RNA-pr); and trypsin-sensitive non-nucleic acid (Sm)
Nucleolar	RNA	Rare; abolished with ribonuclease

* Abbreviations as in Table 3.2.
† LE cell test detects DNA-histone.

mixed connective tissue disease (see below), SLE and Sjögren's syndrome. A nucleolar pattern from staining a single or multiple nucleoli is relatively rare and thought to be particularly indicative of scleroderma (Ritchie, 1970).

In some SLE sera the diffuse nuclear pattern disappears with increasing dilution of the serum, and may be replaced by a nucleolar or speckled staining. Other technical factors also affect the staining patterns, so that it is unwise to place undue reliance on their diagnostic significance. Perhaps the most specific staining pattern seen in SLE is one described as peripheral (or membranous) staining of nuclei, especially if accompanied by a 'rocket' appearance, which is said to correlate well with the presence of anti-DNA antibody in the serum. The antigens thought to be involved in producing these different patterns are described in Table 3.1.

Since the techniques used do not usually conform to a standardized method, and different substrates are used, it is not surprising that strict comparisons cannot be made between published series. For example, the use of peripheral leucocytes as a substrate is associated with a very high incidence of a class of anti-nuclear antibodies which are more typical of rheumatoid arthritis. Other substrates which have been used include nucleated chicken red cells rich in DNA and the organism *Crithidia luciliae* (a protozoon) which possesses a kinetoplast rich in DS-DNA, and positive tests apparently correlate well with the Farr binding assay. Immunofluorescent tests are of established value in screening procedures, but are not sufficiently specific or quantifiable for accurate clinical diagnosis or sequential studies.

ANTIBODY TO DEFINED NUCLEAR AND CYTOPLASMIC ANTIGENS (Table 3.2)

1. *Antibodies to DNA*

Antibodies to deoxyribonucleic acid (DNA), both in a double strand (DS) structure and single strand form (SS), are described. Many different methods for the detection of antibodies to various nuclear (and cytoplasmic) antigens are in use. Techniques which employ precipitation in agar, complement fixation, haemagglutination, or agglutination of latex or bentonite particles coated with nucleic

Table 3.2 Clinical significance of antibodies to nuclear and cytoplasmic antigens

Antigen	Abbreviation	Disease association*
Nuclear		
Deoxyribonucleoprotein	DNA-Pr	As for LE cells and homogeneous anti-nuclear antibody
Double-stranded deoxyribonucleic acid	DS-DNA	SLE, especially active disease
Single-stranded deoxyribonucleic acid	SS-DNA	SLE, RA, SS, CAH, PBC
Extractable nuclear antigen	ENA	MCTD, PM, SC, SLE, SS
Soluble, non-nucleic acid molecule	Sm†	SLE
Ribonucleoprotein	RNA-Pr (? same as Mo)	MCTD, SLE
Cytoplasmic		
Ribosomes	—	SLE
Mitochondria	—	PBC, CAH
Ribonucleoprotein	La	As for RNA-Pr above
Soluble non-nucleic acid	Ro	SLE, SS

* Only common associations are mentioned and, if more than one, in order of frequency.
Abbreviations: CAH, chronic active hepatitis; MCTD, mixed connective tissue disease; PBC, primary biliary cirrhosis; PM, polymyositis; RA, rheumatoid arthritis; SC, scleroderma; SLE, systemic lupus erythematosus; SS, Sjögren's syndrome.
† Sm, Mo, La and Ro are named after patients in whose sera antibodies were first described; Sm and Ro are antigenically dissimilar.

acids, are considered to be less sensitive than assays which employ radio-labelled antigens in primary binding assays, for example, employing the technique described by Farr (1958). The purest form of radio-labelled DS-DNA is probably obtained by internal labelling and an extraction procedure which eliminates other contaminating nucleic acids and proteins. However, the molecular weight of the DNA is not usually controlled and neither is its shape (e.g. circular for bacteriophage DS-DNA and linear for other forms of mammalian DNA), and both influence antibody-binding capacity. The antigenic nature of nucleic acids is reviewed by Stollar (1973).

Antibodies to SS-DNA occur in a variety of diseases, including SLE and rheumatoid arthritis (Koffler *et al.*, 1971). Antibodies to DS-DNA are diagnostically more specific for SLE and raised levels usually reflect disease activity (Schur and Sandson, 1968; Holian *et al.*, 1975). Even so, low levels of antibodies to DS-DNA have been described in normal healthy individuals, although DNA binding to non-immunoglobulin molecules occurs, and proof of the immuno-globulin nature of the binding reactions is not usually sought. The occurrence and clinical significance of raised levels of antibodies to DS-DNA and SS-DNA are tabulated in Table 3.2.

2. *Antibodies to DNA-histone*

Antibodies directed against DNA-histone are responsible for the LE cell pheno-mena and correspond to the common anti-nuclear antibody detected by im-munofluorescence (see Table 3.1).

3. *Antibodies to 'extractable nuclear antigens' (non-DNA)*

A composite antigen containing nuclear RNA-protein and non-nucleic acid (SM) antigens (corresponding to that detected by speckled staining) is obtained by using a phosphate-buffer-saline extract of nuclei and is termed 'extractable nuclear antigens' (ENA) and antibodies to this extract are detected in patients with SLE and 'mixed connective tissue disease' (Sharp *et al.*, 1971). Antibodies to RNAse sensitive component of ENA are thought to be particularly charac-teristic of a disease syndrome of arthritis with some features of scleroderma and polymyositis. This syndrome, termed 'mixed connective tissue disease' is how-ever not distinctive enough clinically to be easily separable from systemic lupus without renal involvement, and certain patients with scleroderma and poly-myositis with multi-system manifestations. However, its recognition is claimed to be of some significance since these patients are very responsive to small doses of steroids and have a good prognosis. Antibodies to Sm are confined to SLE patients who show the more classical clinical picture (Tan and Kunkel, 1966).

4. *Antibodies to nucleolar components and RNA*

Separated nucleoli have been employed in tests and give reactions similar to those that are detected by immunofluorescence. The finding of uracil-specific anti-RNA antibodies in all scleroderma patients may be relevant to this obser-vation (Alarcon-Segovia and Fishbin, 1975). Antibodies to double-stranded synthetic RNA and reovirus have been described in the sera of patients with SLE and have led to the speculation that an RNA-type virus may be implicated in patients with SLE in the manner similar to that seen in New Zealand mice (Chapter 6).

5. *Antibodies to other nuclear and cytoplasmic antigens*

See Table 3.2 for antibodies to other antigens.

HETEROGENEITY

The results of investigations of anti-nuclear antibodies (ANA) have suggested that all classes of immunoglubolin are represented in individual sera; namely, IgG, IgM and IgA. (IgG antibodies correlate with the occurrence of LE cells, whereas IgM anti-nuclear antibodies do not and are diagnostically less specific.) The finding of various nuclear antigens and anti-nuclear antibodies in serum and eluates of kidneys of patients with SLE indicates that many of them might be involved in any single patient in the production of immune-complex-mediated renal damage (Koffler *et al.*, 1974).

Two other properties of anti-DNA antibody are probably of pathogenetic importance.

1. Antibodies which precipitate with DS-DNA using the technique of immunoelectrophoresis correlate with the occurrence of vasculitis in SLE (as well as a few patients with rheumatoid arthritis) (Johnson *et al.*, 1973).

2. The rate of dissociation between DNA and anti-DNA antibody has been shown to differ between patients with and without renal lupus (Steward *et al.*, 1974).

Cellular Immunity to Autoantigens

Recent studies have investigated the role of cellular immunity to autoantigens in rheumatoid arthritis, SLE, Sjögren's syndrome, polymyositis and polymyalgia rheumatica (Table 3.3).

Reactions to IgG

Using lymphocyte transformation tests, results of studies in rheumatoid arthritis have not been consistent (Table 3.3). In general, no stimulation of lymphocytes has been observed, although in one study using autologous serum as supplement, aggregated IgG was stimulatory. Autologous IgG was similarly stimulatory in another study. Skin reactions to IgG of Arthus type have been noted but are not increased in rheumatoid patients. However, in direct migration of leucocytes from capillary tubes into culture chambers, IgG (native or aggregated) was found to inhibit rheumatoid leucocytes more than controls. In tests on supernatants derived from lymphocytes stimulated with IgG, MIF-like activity was found from patients with rheumatoid arthritis (Table 3.3).

Reactions to synovial cells

The possibility that changes in rheumatoid synovium are a result of allergic reactions to an antigen that might be present in rheumatoid connective tissue cells has been investigated (Table 3.3). The presence of circulating sensitized lymphocytes to such antigens in rheumatoid patients was believed to be the basis of cytotoxic effects on a human fibroblastic cell line *in vitro* (Hedberg and Källen, 1964); however, the fibroblast cells would be expected to possess distinct HL-A or other genetically determined antigenic differences which could account for these results. Moreover, the experiments could not be repeated in other laboratories. More recently, it has been reported that fibroblast-like synovial cell lines derived from rheumatoid and normal subjects were both shown to be liable to

Table 3.3 Cellular immunity to autoantigens

Disease	Antigen	Cell-mediated immunity test	Result	Disease vs Control	Reference
RA	IgG (native or aggregated)	LT	Negative	Same	Kackaki *et al.,* 1969
	Agg IgG (+ autoserum)	LT	Positive	Increased	Kinsella, 1974
	Auto-IgG, IgM	LT	Positive	Increased	Dorner *et al.,* 1974
	IgG (native or aggregated)	LMT	Positive	Increased	Froland & Gaarder, 1973
	IgG	MIF	Positive	Increased	Sany *et al.,* 1975
	IgG	DH	Negative	Same	Chamberlain *et al.,* 1970
	Synovial membrane	LMT	Positive	Increased	Bacon *et al.,* 1973
			Negative	Same	Panayi, 1976
	Synovial cell line	LMT	Negative	Same	Marsh *et al.,* 1975
SLE	DNA	LT	Positive	Increased	Goldman *et al.,* 1972
		LMT	Positive	Decreased	Federlin & Helmke, 1972
		MIF	Positive	Increased	Abe *et al.,* 1973
		DH	Positive	Increased	Goldman *et al.,* 1972
Sjögren's syndrome	Salivary gland	LMT	Positive	Increased	Soborg & Bertrom, 1968
Polymyositis	Muscle	LT	Positive	Increased	Chapter 8
		LCTX	Positive	Increased	
		LTXN	Positive	Increased	
Polymyalgia rheumatica	Muscle	LT	Positive	Increased	Esiri *et al.,* 1973
	Arterial extract	LT	Positive	Increased	Hazelman *et al.,* 1975

Abbreviations: DH, delayed hypersensitivity; LCTX, lymphocyte cytotoxicity; LMT, leucocyte migration test; LT, lymphocyte transformation; LTXN, lymphotoxin; MIF, migration inhibition factor activity.

cytopathic effects when exposed to rheumatoid leucocytes, although the effects were most marked when rheumatoid cell line and leucocyte combinations were used. These results suggest that a population of rheumatoid lymphocytes unique to the disease react with antigens which are best expressed on the surface of rheumatoid synovial cells. The use of an extract of rheumatoid synovial membrane as antigen in the leucocyte migration test was also taken to indicate the presence of lymphocytes sensitized to synovial antigens (Bacon *et al.*, 1973). The possibility that this result may have been due to surface-absorbed immunoglobulin in a manner similar to that observed when Mycoplasma antigens are used in leucocyte migration tests has to be excluded (Chapter 5). The possibility that synovial cells may express virus-coded antigens on their surface, and thereby overcome tolerance to autoantigens and lead to the production of autoimmune reactions, remains an interesting theoretical possibility (Chapter 1).

Reactions to other antigens

Cellular immunity to DNA has been assessed by a variety of tests with inconclusive results (Table 3.3). Using supernatants of lymphocytes cultured with DNA, migration inhibition factor has been demonstrated. In the direct leucocyte migration test (LMT), for inexplicable reasons, LMT on SLE patients showed little or no inhibition whilst most healthy control subjects were positive. Positive lymphocyte transformation tests with DNA have been reported. Several authors have claimed positive delayed hypersensitivity reactions to DNA in patients with SLE, whilst in another study such reactions were rare and could not be differentiated from those occurring in controls.

Other antigenic preparations which showed positive reactions in one or other test of cellular immunity include salivary gland extracts in Sjögren's syndrome, muscle antigens in polymyositis and polymyalgia rheumatica and arterial extracts in polymyalgia rheumatica.

References

ABE, T., HARA, M., YAMASAKI, K. and HOMMA, M. (1973). *Arthr. and Rheum.*, **16**, 688.

ALARCON-SEGOVIA, D. and FISHBIN, E. (1975). *Lancet*, **1**, 363.

BACON, P. A., CRACCHIOLO, A., BLUESTONE, R. and GOLDBERG, L. S. (1973). *Lancet*, **2**, 699.

BARTFIELD, M. D. (1969). *Ann. N.Y. Acad. Sci.*, **168**, 30.

BIANCO, N. E., DOBKIN, L. W. and SCHUR, P. H. (1974). *Clin. exp. Immunol.*, **17**, 91.

CALCOTT, M. A. and MULLER-EBERHARD, H. J. (1972). *Biochemistry*, **11**, 3443.

CAPRA, J. D., WINCHESTER, R. J. and KUNKEL, H. G. (1971). *Medicine (Baltimore)*, **50**, 125.

CHAMBERLAIN, M. A., SHAPLAND, C. G. and ROITT, I. M. (1970). *Ann. rheum. Dis.*, **29**, 173.

DORNER, R. W., GANTNER, G. E., GOLDSCHMIDT, J., ZUCKNER, J. and FUDENBERG, H. H. (1974). *Immunology*, **27**, 781.

ESIRI, M. M., MACLENNAN, I. M. and HAZELMAN, B. L. (1973). *Clin. exp. Immunol.*, **14**, 25.

FARR, R. S. (1958). *J. infect. Dis.*, **103**, 239.

FEDERLIN, K. and HELMKE, K. (1972). *Lancet*, **1**, 596.

FEHR, K., VELVART, M. and BOENI, A. (1975). *Scand. J. Rheumatol.*, Suppl. 8, 25.

FELL, H. B. and BARRATT, M. E. J. (1973). *Int. Arch. Allergy. appl. Immunol.*, **44**, 441.

FROLAND, S. S. and GAARDER, P. I. (1973). *Scand. J. Immunol.*, **2**, 385.

GOLDMAN, J. A., LITWIN, A., ADAMS, L. E., KRUEGGER, R. C. and HESS, E. V. (1972). *J. clin. Invest.*, **51**, 2669.

HARRIS, J. and VAUGHAN, J. H. (1961). *Arthr. and Rheum.*, **4**, 47.

HAZELMAN, B. L., MACLENNAN, I. C. M. and ESIRI, M. M. (1975). *Ann. rheum. Dis.*, **34**, 122.

HEDBERG, H. and KÄLLEN, B. D. (1964). *Acta path. microbiol. scand.*, **62**, 177.

HOLIAN, J., GRIFFITHS, I. D., GLASS, D. N., MAINI, R. N. and SCOTT, J. T. (1975). *Ann. rheum. Dis.* **34**, 438.

HOWELL, F. A., CHAMBERLAIN, M. A., PERRY, R. A., TORRIGIANI, G. and ROITT, I. M. (1972). *Ann. rheum. Dis.*, **31**, 129.

JASIN, H. E., LOSPALLUTO, J. and ZIFF, M. (1970). *Amer. J. Med.*, **49**, 484.

JOHNSON, G. D., EDMONDS, J. P. and HOLBOROW, E. J. (1973). *Lancet*, **2**, 883.

KACKAKI, J., BULLOCK, W. and VAUGHAN, J. (1969). *Lancet*, **1**, 1289.

KINSELLA, T. (1974). *J. clin. Invest.*, **53**, 1108.

KOFFLER, D., CARR, R., AGNELLO, V., THOBURN, R. and KUNKEL, H. G. (1971). *J. exp. Med.*, **134**, 294.

KOFFLER, D., AGNELLO, V. and KUNKEL, H. G. (1974). *Amer. J. Path.*, **74**, 109.

KULKA, J. P. (1959). *J. chron. Dis.*, **10**, 388.

KUNKEL, H. G. and TAN, E. (1964). *Adv. Immunol.*, **4**, 351.

LOSPALLUTO, J., FEHR, K. and ZIFF, M. (1970). *J. Immunol.*, **105**, 886.

MARSH, J. M., ROFFE, L. M. and MAINI, R. N. (1975). Unpublished.

MELLBYE, O. I. and NATVIG, J. B. (1971). *Clin. exp. Immunol.*, **8**, 889.

MELTZER, M. and FRANKLIN, E. C. (1966). *Amer. J. Med.*, **40**, 828.

MILLROY, S. J. and POOLE, A. R. (1974). *Ann. rheum. Dis.*, **33**, 500.

MUNTHE, E. and NATVIG, J. B. (1971). *Clin. exp. Immunol.*, **8**, 249.

NATVIG, J. B., MUNTHE, E. and GAARDER, P. I. (1971). In *Rheumatoid Arthritis*, p. 343. Ed. W. Muller, H. G. Harwerth and K. Fehr. Academic Press, New York and London.

NATVIG, J. B., GAARDER, P. I. and TURNER, M. W. (1972). *Clin. exp. Immunol.*, **12**, 177.

NATVIG, J. B., MUNTHE, E. and PAHLE, J. (1975). *Rheumatology*, **6**, 167.

NOTKINS, A. L. (1971). *J. exp. Med.*, **134**, 32 (s).

PANAYI, G. (1976). *Ann. rheum. Dis.* (abstr) (in press).

PANUSH, R. S., BIANCO, N. E. and SCHUR, P. H. (1971). *Arthur. and Rheum.*, **14**, 737.

POOLE, A. R., BARRATT, M. E. J. and FELL, H. B. (1973). *Int. Arch. Allergy. appl. Immunol.*, **44**, 469.

RAWSON, A. J., QUISMORIO, F. P. and ABELSON, N. M. (1969). *Amer. J. Path.*, **54**, 95.

RITCHIE, R. F. (1970). *New Engl. J. Med.*, **282**, 1174.

SANY, J., MATHIEU, O., CLOT, J., MANDIN, J. and SERRE, H. (1975). *Rheumatology*, **6**, 131.

SCHUR, P. H. and SANDSON, J. (1968). *New Engl. J. Med.*, **278**, 533.

SHARP, G. C., IRVIN, W. S., LAROQUE, R. L., VELEZ, C., DALY, V., KAISER, A. D. and HOLMAN, H. R. (1971). *J. clin. Invest.*, **50**, 350.

SOBORG, M. and BERTROM, U. (1968). *Acta med. scand.*, **184**, 319.

STEFFEN, C. (1971). In *Rheumatoid Arthritis*, p. 411. Ed. W. Muller, H. G. Harweth and K. Fehr. Academic Press, New York and London.

STEWARD, M. W., GLASS, D. N., MAINI, R. N. and SCOTT, J. T. (1974). *J. Rheumatol.*, **1** (suppl. 1), 41.

STOLLAR, B. D. (1973). In *The Antigens*, Vol. 1, p. 1. Ed. M. Sela. Academic Press, New York and London.

TAN, E. M. and KUNKEL, H. G. (1966). *J. Immunol.*, **96**, 464.

WINCHESTER, R. J., AGNELLO, V. and KUNKEL, H. G. (1969). *Arthr. and Rheum.*, **12**, 343.

WINCHESTER, R. J., AGNELLO, V. and KUNKEL, H. G. (1970). *Clin. exp. Immunol.*, **6**, 689.

4

Immunological Methods

A number of methods and techniques have been employed in the investigation of immunological processes involved in rheumatic diseases. The principles and background of a few are described in this section on the basis of their extensive current application and relevance to rheumatic diseases, whilst some others are covered in other chapters (e.g. autoantibodies) but many remain beyond the scope of this book (see the Reference, 'Immunological Methods' for a list of suitable books and manuals).

Studies on fresh tissues

SOURCE OF MATERIAL

Surgical procedures on affected joints (e.g. synovectomy in rheumatoid arthritis and menisectomy in traumatized knee joints of otherwise healthy individuals) have provided a source of fresh material. Although the amount of tissue is usually considerable, and this may be desirable, surgery is often undertaken long after the onset of disease, by which time pathological changes may not be relevant to the process under investigation. The use of techniques of percutaneous biopsy of the synovium under local anaesthesia not only allows the procedure to be undertaken early in the course of the disease, but, when obtained under direct vision at the time of arthroscopy, permits examination of selective and multiple biopsies. Furthermore, it is possible to repeat the procedure on a subsequent occasion.

Skin and muscle specimens are usually obtained by excision biopsy, care being taken to avoid trauma to the tissues so as not to distort them for microscopical studies. Since such incisions leave scars it may not be practicable to repeat them very often, and for the purposes of repeated studies 'punch' needle biopsies may be employed, but may distort the tissue. The use of percutaneous renal biopsies (e.g. in systemic lupus erythematosus), percutaneous liver biopsies (e.g. in auto-immune hepatitis) and rectal biopsies through a sigmoidoscope (for amyloid deposit in blood vessel wall) have contributed significantly to the understanding of the immunology of rheumatic diseases.

MICROSCOPY

Tissue sections obtained by the methods detailed above have been examined in a variety of ways for changes relevant to immune pathogenesis. For example, using ordinary light microscopy, the distribution and organization of immune cells in conventionally stained sections may indirectly indicate their participation in immunological, inflammatory or tissue-damaging reactions. Thus, perivascular cuffing with lymphocytes indicates a pathological process in which increased vascular permeability is associated with cellular emigration into tissues. Germinal centre formation and proliferation of plasma cells at the cortico-medullary junction and medulla in lymph nodes indicate a B cell response to antigen challenge, whilst cellular accumulation and proliferation in paracortical areas indicate a T cell response. Germinal centre formation and lymphocyte aggregates in perivascular areas in rheumatoid synovium could therefore be interpreted as representing a B cell response to antigen associated with increased vascular permeability, a concept of some pathogenetic interest. The close proximity of lymphocytes to necrotic muscle fibres in polymyositis or liver cells in chronic aggressive hepatitis could indicate their possible role in producing tissue damage. Further characterization of immune cells may be undertaken by examining histochemical characteristics (e.g. using vital stains such as acridine orange or euchrysine which stain lysosomal enzymes of histocytes in macrophages); or demonstration of intracytoplasmic antibody by immunofluorescent fluorescein-conjugated antiglobulins indicating synthesized immunoglobulin (e.g. in plasma cells). However, these techniques do not necessarily distinguish between locally synthesized antibody and antibody which has been interiorized by phagocytosis or pinocytosis, the usual criterion of distinction being indirect and based on identification of the morphology of the cell—thus, plasma cells are assumed to have synthesized, and histiocytic cells phagocytosed, antibody.

Examination of finer ultrastructural details by electron microscopy may differentiate between various cell types; for example, the presence of aggregated polyribosomes and nucleoli without endoplasmic reticulum indicates that the cell is probably a lymphoblast, and may distinguish it from plasma cells which are rich in endoplasmic reticulum. The thymic-dependent (T) or bone-marrow-dependent (B) lymphocytes in tissues have been directly demonstrated in fresh tissues by techniques which employ adherence of sheep red cells (E rosettes) to detect T cells, and antibody- or complement-coated red cells (EA and C3 rosettes) for B cells.

The use of fluorescein-conjugated antiglobulin allows localization of extracellular immunoglobulin deposits in tissue sections, and when the sections are also stained for complement components such as C3, the findings are taken to provide evidence for the presence of immune complexes. Rarely is it possible also to stain for antigens, if known in these immune complexes, by using suitably fluorosceinated antibodies. Electron-dense material shown by electron microscopy increases the sensitivity of detection and localization of immune deposits and allows studies of their relationship to adjacent cells and matrix, and has also contributed to the current concept of immune complex tissue damage.

Immunochemistry of tissue fluids and eluates

Characterization of amounts, classes, quality and specificities of antibodies in blood and tissue fluids, as well as eluates of affected tissues, forms the basis of an important method of study which has shed light on pathogenetic mechanisms. Detection of antigens is also sometimes possible, and is assuming great signicance in the detection of infective agents which may be implicated in the aetiology of rheumatic diseases. Studies of complement and immune complexes are discussed below.

Tissue culture

The techniques of tissue culture employing culture media and conditions promoting cell viability *in vitro* have been extensively employed in the investigation of rheumatic diseases and are referred to in this book in various chapters. Using such techniques, cells may be cultured in suspension or monolayers, and pieces of tissue or organs may be maintained for experiments over a short term (lasting hours or days) or long term (lasting several weeks). The considerable body of knowledge that now exists in relation to the function of lymphocytes, antibody-synthesizing cells, mononuclear and polymorphonuclear phagocytes as effector cells, all of which play an important role in rheumatic diseases, has been derived from tissue culture methods. Evidence of infection with viruses or other organisms has been sought by special culture techniques coupled with immunological methods on tissues from patients. For example, specific microbial antigens have been sought on cultured rheumatoid synovial cells by using antisera to known organisms (e.g. rubella) in cytotoxicity and immunofluorescent tests. Attempts at demonstrating the presence of specifically sensitized lymphocytes in patients to extrinsic microbial or intrinsic autoantigens or newly derived antigens (e.g. mutational or as a result of infection) have utilized tests of cellular immunity, such as lymphocyte transformation and cell migration (see later in this chapter).

The technique of culturing pieces of synovium from rheumatoid patients has demonstrated that antibody and lymphokine synthesis is maintained *in vitro*—in the case of the former for up to 30–40 weeks, supporting the important concept of a perpetual local immune response in the synovium, no doubt contributing to the observed chronicity of the disease. Experiments on pieces of salivary tissue in culture have shown that antibodies, including rheumatoid factor, are similarly produced in Sjögren's syndrome. The maintenance of cartilage pieces and limb rudiments in culture together with antibodies to chondrocytes has contributed to an understanding of the breakdown and regeneration processes in cartilage.

Complement

Studies on complement proteins, mechanisms of their activation, their role in generation of phlogistic and tissue-damaging reactions and documentation of changes in blood and affected tissues, as well as in the synovial fluid in joints, have lead to some of the current theories of the immunological pathways involved in tissue damage, particularly in relation to immune complex damage (see Chapter 2). The complement system consists of at least nine component proteins which, following activation, interact and generate biologically active products. At least three inhibitors are also described which can arrest the reactions at various stages (reviewed by Lachmann, 1975). An over-all picture of the integrity of the complement system is obtained by measuring the functional ability of complement to support haemolysis of sheep red cells sensitized with antibody, the result being expressed as CH_{50} units/ml (Schur and Austen, 1971). The same technique has been suitably modified to detect individual components. A reduction in total haemolytic activity is usually taken as evidence of dimunution in the levels of one or more components of the system resulting from activation and consumption of complement. However, in certain circumstances the functional ability of complement may be lowered owing to diminution in the amount of one of the three inhibitors of the reaction. It should also be pointed out that a fall in individual complement proteins does not always indicate consumption; synthesis may be low, in some instances owing to a genetically inherited deficiency.

An important mechanism leading to a fall in complement levels is related to its consumption following activation by immune complexes via the so-called 'classical pathway' (Fig. 4.1). Immune complexes combine with the 'early' components C1, C4 and C2 and lead to the generation of an enzymatic activity capable of cleavage of C3. A similar activity for C3 is also generated by the 'alternate pathway' involving other proteins in blood, namely properdin, factor B (C3PA) and factor D (C3PAse), the initiating stimulus being less characterized and apparently not dependent on immune complexes (Fig. 4.1). In a sense, C3 is pivotal to the activation sequence, lowered levels indicating utilization of

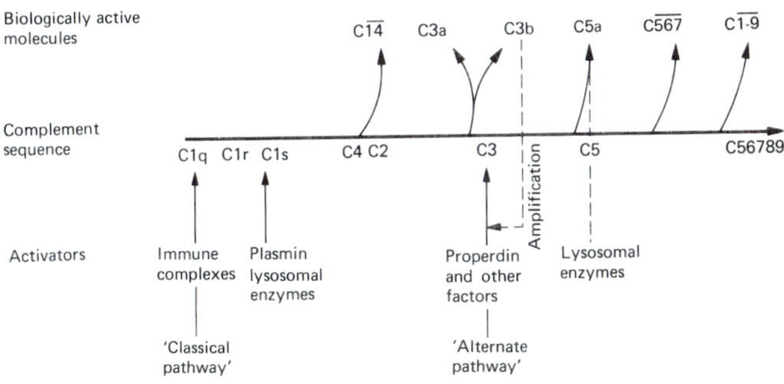

Fig. 4.1   The sequential activation of complement proteins is shown diagrammatically. Activators include immune complexes ('classical pathway'), plasmin, lysosomal enzymes and properdin (and other factors of the 'alternate pathway'). Biologically active molecules are shown and include C14 (virus neutralization), C3a (anaphylotoxin), C3b (concerned with 'immune adherence'), C5a (chemotaxis and anaphylotoxin), C567 (chemotaxis), and C19 (membrane lysis).

complement by either pathway, and usually correlating with reduction in haemolytic activity. If lowered C3 (and haemolytic complement activity) is accompanied by diminution of C1, C4 and C2, the evidence suggests classical pathway activation and indirectly implies that immune complexes were responsible for triggering the reaction, whereas normal levels of these early components with lowered C3 or haemolytic activity favour alternate pathway utilization. More direct evidence of alternate pathway activation may be obtained by showing diminution in properdin or factor B levels. In practice, the tests most often used include haemolytic assays for total haemolytic capacity and detection of individual components, and the use of specific antisera in radial or electro-immunodiffusion tests for detection of C3, C4 and factor B, other complement protein antibodies not being readily available. Inactivation products of C3 and C4 which are antigenetically similar to their parent components, and are therefore reactive with antisera to C3 and C4 but have altered electrophoretic charge, may be detected using a technique of two-dimensional immunoelectrophoresis. The presence of such products indicates complement activation. More recently polyethylene glycol has been used to fractionate the different products of activated C3, C4 and factor B, and, using appropriate antisera in radial immunodiffusion tests, detection of these fragments provides quantitative information on the extent of complement activation (Perrin *et al.*, 1975). The interested reader is referred to a review by Alper (1974) for further background and details on the biology of complement and details of techniques, as well as the precautions that are necessary in interpretation of the data.

Deposition of complement components Clq, C3 and C4 together with immunoglobulin, detected by immunofluorescent techniques applied to frozen tissue sections, provides evidence for immune-complex-mediated tissue damage, the presence of Clq and C4 in this case indicating classical pathway complement activation. More recently, suitable fluoresceinated antisera to properdin and factor B (C3PA) have become available and are used on tissue sections to seek evidence of alternate pathway activation. Interesting patterns of immunofluorescence have been obtained on kidney biopsies of patients with SLE, suggesting that both pathways may be involved. The relative importance of the two pathways, however, remains a subject for future investigation. Furthermore, it is unlikely that the presence of complement components in tissue sections always indicates an immunological initiation; for example, proteolytic enzymes released at sites of tissue damage have been shown to activate C1, C3 and C5.

Measurement of circulating immune complexes

Measurement of circulating complexes (Table 4.1) is a problem central to the investigation of immunologically mediated rheumatic disease. Detection of cryoglobulins and evidence of complement consumption were until recently the only readily available pointers towards the presence of circulating immune complexes. Analytical ultracentrifugation demonstrated the presence of molecules larger than naturally occurring immunoglobulins but little information on their composition. Table 4.1 illustrates the range of assays now being evaluated,

Table 4.1   Methods of detecting immune complexes

Procedure	Technique	Comment	Reference
Physico-chemical methods	Analytical ultracentrifugation	Detects large quantities	Kunkel *et al.*, 1961
	Chromatography	Has to be distinguished from non-complexed Ig Attached C3 detection has been used	Williams & Slaney, 1976
	Density gradient ultracentrifugation	Used in conjunction with sensitive assays for Ig. Most suitable for known antigen-Ab complex	Bombardieri *et al.*, 1973
	Salt precipitation, and double-antibody precipitation	Suitable for known antigens (either labelled with isotope or detectable by other reactions, usually with antisera)	
	Cryoprecipitates	Proteins other than Ig precipitate; may detect special type of complex	Meltzer & Franklin, 1966
	Polyethylene glycol (PEG) precipitation	At appropriate concentrations precipitates complexes	Creighton *et al.*, 1973
Binding of complexes to complement components	C1q fixation in gel	C1q will bind to medium to large complexes	Agnello *et al.*, 1970
	^{125}I-C1q fixation	Also binds to other macro-molecules (e.g. DNA) ? how common	Nyedegger *et al.*, 1974
	Anti-complementary activity	? Relationship to others	Johnson *et al.*, 1975
Binding to rheumatoid factor	Precipitation in 'gel'	Precipitates complexes which do not react with C1q	Winchester *et al.*, 1971
Cell receptor binding	Guinea-pig macrophages	Displacement of isotope-labelled aggregated IgG from Fc receptors	Onyewotu *et al.*, 1974
	Raji cell assay	Reaction with C and Fc receptors on lympho-blastoid cell line	Theofilopoulous *et al.*, 1974
	K cell cytotoxicity	Complexes inhibit K cell killing by binding to Fc receptor on K cells	MacLennan, 1972
	Platelet aggregation	Detects small complexes and those formed at equivalence (Fc receptor reaction)	Penttinen *et al.*, 1971
Others	Electronmicroscopy	Viral material (e.g. hepatitis B)	Almeida, 1971
	Inhibition of IgG-coated latex agglutination	Rheumatoid factor and C1q agglutinate, complexes compete and inhibit reaction	Lurhuma *et al.*, 1976
	Histamine release	Bioassay on quinea-pig lung : tedious	Baumal & Border, 1968
	Detection of antigen and antibody	Reaction of same or sequential serum with antibody and defined antigen (e.g. DNA, anti-DNA)	

the very multiplicity suggesting uncertainty as to specificity, since in the majority the antigen and antibody combination is not identified as such. The assays utilize various physical and biological properties of complexes, including the ability to fix complement. The latter leads to a major difficulty since the presence of functionally active complement in the fresh sera to be assayed competes and interferes with the test, whilst heating sera to 56°C to effect removal of complement is likely to produce aggregation of gammaglobulin, which resembles immune complexes in biological activity.

Tests of cellular immunity

The role of cellular immune mechanisms in rheumatic diseases is still not well defined. Techniques which allow identification of classes of lymphocytes in blood and synovial fluid, as well as measurement of the functional capacity of the lymphocytes, are being increasingly investigated. The techniques include documentation of naturally acquired delayed hypersensitivity to microbial antigens, and the quantification of the degree of sensitization that is produced by contact sensitizing agents such as dinitrochlorobenzene (DNCB), as well as antigens to which patients are unlikely to have come across previously, for example, keyhole limpet haemocyanin (KLH). A number of *in vitro* tests of cellular immunity are being assessed and the techniques employed widely include lymphocyte transformation, leucocyte migration inhibition and measurement of products of activated lymphocytes (for example, migration inhibition factor). Non-antibody mediators generated by activated lymphocytes (lymphokines) and pre-formed material extracted from sensitized lymphocytes (transfer factors) are under active investigation. The general concept has emerged that cellular immunity in patients with a number of different connective tissue diseases is impaired; this may be one of the factors leading to persistence of extrinsic antigens and exaggeration of the humoral response.

Heterogeneity of lymphoid cells in man is definable in terms of: morphology; histochemistry; cell density; electrostatic charge; surface immunoglobulin synthesized by the cell; receptor sites on lymphocyte membranes for the Fc part of Ig, C3 component of complement, and theta or other antigens specific for thymocytes; binding to sheep erythrocytes; capacity to adhere to glass and Nylon; and ability to phagocytose. These characteristics have been utilized to define and enumerate subpopulations of lymphoid cells. However, it has become recognized that methodological details and reagents have varied so considerably from one laboratory to another that even when seemingly similar techniques are used, gross differences and discrepancies are found. It is not clear to what extent separation and purification procedures such as density gradients and passage through columns containing beads, Nylon, etc., lead to selective and variable losses of one or more types of cells, and make the end-product unrepresentative of the starting material.

With regard to surface Ig, the hallmark of a B cell, difficulties arise in distinguishing between secreted Ig and external Ig which has become attached to the lymphocyte membrane. Lymphocyte membranes with receptors for the Fc portion of immunoglobulin may pick up any aggregated IgG from the tissue culture medium. Furthermore, the serum of the lymphocyte donor (particularly in rheumatic diseases) may contain immune complexes which also bind to Fc receptors, or anti-lymphocyte antibodies directed against lymphocyte antigenic determinants which bind to a great proportion of lymphocytes. Winchester *et al.* (1974) have drawn attention to the observation that incubation of lymphocytes in sera at 4°C from patients with rheumatoid arthritis and SLE, leads to acquisition of surface immunoglobulin by as many as 90 per cent of mononuclear cells, possibly due to the presence of cold-reactive anti-lymphocyte antibodies. Some of the Ig-positive cells in peripheral blood from such patients may therefore represent such an artefact.

The normal distribution and occurrence of many other receptors is also uncertain at present. Fc receptors, for example, may be present on a variety of cell types, such as cells which also possess surface Ig and receptors for C3 (typical B cells); or be present in the absence of surface Ig, or in varying combinations. Furthermore, immature or differentiated cells may not express their surface characteristics fully (for example, plasma cells do not have surface Ig). Activated cells, on the other hand, may acquire new surface characteristics; for example, activated T cells may have Fc receptors. All these factors have no doubt contributed to a certain degree of confusion and the lack of agreement so evident in published literature.

Lymphocyte function tests also lack proper standardization and have not been suitably quantified. In many instances the biological basis of the tests remains controversial; for example, in terms of whether B cells or T cells, or both, are stimulated, and whether co-operation of monocytes (or macrophages) is necessary. Repeated sequential tests on the same individual vary enormously, and it is not established whether this arises as a result of technical variations or whether it represents a genuine fluctuation in lymphocyte biology. A bewildering variety of modifications of the same test is sometimes evident. For example, lymphocyte transformation can be undertaken on whole blood, leucocytes and on preparations of lymphocytes of varying degrees of purity, in a variety of culture media, with different types of serum supplements and different grades of chemically defined mitogens and antigens (carrying the same name). The dose-response and time-course of such tests vary with the antigen or mitogen, and perhaps even between healthy individuals.

Attempts at achieving a classification of lymphoid cells in terms of surface characteristics are described below (Table 4.2). The following classes are recognized: (1) T cells; (2) B cells; (3) K cells; and (4) monocytes (or macrophages). For more detailed information see reviews by Froland and Natvig (1973), Jondal *et al.* (1973), Nussenzweig (1974), Warner (1974), and a WHO/IARC-sponsored Workshop report (1974). For tests of lymphocyte function see the Reference, 'In vitro methods in cell-mediated immunity: a progress report' (1973).

The following methods have been utilized to characterize lymphocytes and cellular immune reactions (Table 4.2).

Table 4.2   Cell surface and functional characteristics of lymphocyte subpopulations and monocytes

Cell surface and other characteristics		T	B	K	Mono/Macro	Test used*
1. Sheep erythrocyte binding		+	−	−	−	E-rosette
2. T-cell-specific antigens (e.g. theta, θ)		+	−	−	−	Fl. or cytotoxic T antisera
3. Surface immunoglobulin (secreted by cell)		−	+	−	−	Fl. anti-Ig antisera
4. Fc receptor		−(?)	+	+	+	Fl. agg. Ig ; EA rosette
5. C3 receptor		−	+	?	+	EAC rosette
6. Adherence to glass		−	−	−	+	Column ; petri dish
7. Nylon adherence		−	+	−	+	Column
8. Enzymes rich in phagocytes		−	−	−	+	Euchrysine or peroxidase staining
9. Ab-dependent cytotoxicity		−	−	+	+	Target cell coated with antibody
10. Specific cell–cell cytotoxicity		+	−	−	−	
11. Delayed hypersensitivity		+	−	−	−	Skin tests with antigens read at 48 hours
12. Lymphocyte transformation						
Phytohaemagglutinin	(PHA)	+	?			Usually measured by uptake of
Pokeweed mitogen	(PWM)	+(?)	+			^{3}H-thymidine
Antigen	(Ag)	+	?			
Mixed leucocyte reaction	(MLR)	+	−			'Responder' cell function
Lipopolysaccharide	(LPS)	−	+			
13. Lymphokine production ; e.g.						
mitogenic factor	(MF)	+	−?			^{3}H-thymidine uptake by lymphocytes
Migration inhibition factor	(MIF)	+	+?			Inhibition of macrophage migration

* Abbreviations : A, antibody ; agg., aggregated ; C, complement ; E, erythrocyte ; Fl., fluorescein ; Ig. immunoglobulin.

1. SHEEP ERYTHROCYTE ROSETTES

Sheep erythrocytes form rosettes with thymus-derived T lymphocytes, the lymphocytes being termed 'E-rosette forming cells' (E-Rc). The numbers in normal peripheral blood have been variously estimated between 40 and 90 per cent, the technical conditions presumably being largely responsible for such a wide range. Variables in the technique include temperature and duration of incubation, exclusion of monocytes from counts of total lymphocytes, the ratio of sheep erythrocytes to human lymphocytes used to define a rosette, variability between batches of sheep erythrocytes, presence of serum factors, and pre-treatment with trypsin or other enzymes.

2. ANTISERA AGAINST T CELLS

Antisera against T cells have been raised by immunizing rabbits with human fetal thymocytes and absorbing the serum with B-lymphocyte leukaemia cells, although the specificity of the antisera remains questionable. Anti-lymphocyte antibodies found in certain human sera have also been used for this purpose.

3. SURFACE IMMUNOGLOBULIN

Fluoresceinated anti-human globulin has been utilized to detect surface immunoglobulin on human lymphocytes and, when secreted by the lymphocyte, is regarded as a hallmark of B cells. Using whole antisera against human immunoglobulin, about 20 per cent of the peripheral blood mononuclear cells in healthy individuals show membrane immunofluorescence (reviewed by Warner, 1974). Monospecific antisera have been used to detect the various immunoglobulin classes represented, and results indicate that the largest proportion of cells stain for IgG; IgM, IgA and IgD occur in decreasing frequency. However, in recent studies by Winchester *et al.* (1975), using fluoresceinated pepsin-digested antisera (containing $F(ab^1)_2$ portion of antisera to Ig) less than 10 per cent of the total peripheral blood lymphocytes in normal individuals showed staining for surface immunoglobulin, and using the appropriate class-specific antisera the surprising finding was reported that the majority of Ig-positive cells have specificity for both IgM and IgD.

4. SURFACE COMPLEMENT (C3) RECEPTOR

Erythrocytes coated with specific antibody (IgM should be preferentially used) and complement component C3, form rosettes (termed 'EAC rosettes') with lymphocytes which possess receptors for C3. However, not all Ig-positive cells possess C3 receptors and certain lymphocytes without surface Ig have C3 receptors, usually in conjunction with a receptor for Fc. Although susceptible to trypsin, as is surface Ig, present on the same cell, the complement receptor appears to be a distinct and separate entity. C3 receptors are also detectable on monocytes (see Table 4.1) and granulocytes. These stable receptor sites have to be distinguished from activated C3 which is membrane bound during functional activation of the pathway that leads to lysis of antibody-coated cells (Nussenzweig, 1974).

5. SURFACE FC RECEPTOR

Certain populations of Ig-positive or Ig-negative lymphocytes, monocytes (and macrophages) and polymorphs possess a surface receptor which binds the Fc portion of the heavy chain of immunoglobulin. The Fc portion of aggregated or 'complexed' immunoglobulin molecules bind to the receptor most efficiently. Fc receptors are detected by binding of erythrocytes sensitized with antibody (EA rosettes) or fluoresceinated aggregated IgG. The source of the erythrocytes and the class (or subclass) of antibody, however, appear to determine the number and type of mononuclear cells which bind them, probably because of varying affinity and specificity of the receptor for the Fc part of immunoglobulin. Thus, macrophages (and monocytes) seem to bind IgG1 and IgG3 subclasses exclusively. Using human erythrocytes coated with human anti-CD IgG antibody it has been shown that EA rosettes detect monocytes and a subpopulation of lymphocytes which are surface Ig negative and do not form E-rosettes (about 10 per cent of total lymphocytes in healthy subjects). If ox red cells coated with rabbit anti-ox antibody are used, up to 26 per cent of peripheral blood lymphocytes form rosettes. The use of sheep erythrocytes coated with antibody should be avoided since the unique affinity for T cells of the unsensitized cells cannot be excluded. Aggregated IgG also binds to Fc receptors and, although originally regarded as an alternative method for detecting surface Ig-bearing B cells, it is likely that it also detects subpopulations similar to those reacting with EA systems.

6. GLASS ADHERENCE

Incubation of mononuclear cell suspensions on glass surfaces will lead to adherence of monocytes, and the method may be utilized either to deplete a lymphocyte population of monocytes, or to prepare a pure monocyte population. It is not clear, however, whether all monocytes are adherent.

7. NYLON-FIBRE AND ANTIBODY-COATED COLUMNS

Provided that the Nylon-fibre column is packed in an appropriate fashion, mononuclear cell suspensions passed through these lead to retention of monocytes and a large proportion of B cells. Columns containing Sephadex coated with anti-human-Fab have also been used to deplete B cells. These methods are utilized to obtain pure populations of T cells.

8. STAINING OF CYTOPLASM FOR ENZYMES

Using euchrysine or enzymes such as peroxidase, the cytoplasm of phagocytic cells shows characteristic staining; this method provides a means of differentiating between monocytes and lymphocytes, since only the former are rich in lysosomal enzymes.

9 & 10. CELL-MEDIATED CYTOTOXICITY

The conditions under which K and T cells exert cytotoxicity on target cells have already been described (see Chapter 2). The function or behaviour of the cells has been used as a characteristic of the class of cell participating in the reaction. Thus K cells mediate damage to antibody-coated target cells, and T cells damage target cells for which they are specifically sensitized. It is important to note that although efforts at characterizing K cells in terms of morphology, surface markers and glass adherence have been attempted, the phenomenon of K cell activity is not peculiar to a particular class of cells, since it may be mediated by other Fc-receptor-bearing cells such as monocytes, macrophages and polymorphs.

11. DELAYED HYPERSENSITIVITY

Forty-eight-hour skin reactions at sites of intracutaneous injections of antigens may give rise to an indurated and erythematous reactions (delayed hyper-sensitivity). Although generally regarded as being indicative of T cell sensitization to that antigen, the reaction may be easily confused with a persistent Arthus reaction. Moreover, lymphocyte infiltration of a biopsy site of the reaction is also not diagnostic of T cell reactions since B cells also accumulate at sites of cutaneous reactions, especially in the Jones–Motes reaction.

12. LYMPHOCYTE TRANSFORMATION

Lymphocyte transformation with phytohaemagglutinin (PHA) has been regarded as an exclusive feature of T cell activity although other workers claim that B cells obtained by depletion of T cells also transform with soluble PHA.

Pokeweed mitogen (PWM) is a B cell mitogen but requires T helper cell function, so that *in vitro* transformation with this agent measures B and T cell activity. Mixed leucocyte reactions in which lymphocytes of an individual are stimulated in lymphocyte transformation tests using irradiated or mitomycin-treated lymphocytes as 'stimulator' cells apparently reflect T cell stimulation. Lipopolysaccharide (LPS) is a pure B cell mitogen in mice and does not require T helper function. Whether it is similarly reactive in humans has not been confirmed. Tuberculin PPD and other antigens probably activate T and B cells.

13. LYMPHOKINE PRODUCTION

Culture supernatants from lymphocytes stimulated with antigens or phyto-mitogens possess a number of biological activities relevant to the expression of cellular immunity. These factors, termed 'lymphokines', are non-antibody molecules and may be assayed in a number of ways. Two activities are mentioned, mitogenetic factor which describes the property of increased DNA synthesis in allogeneic or autologous lymphocytes, and migration inhibition factor (MIF) which describes their property of inhibiting migration of guinea-pig macrophages from capillary tubes into tissue culture chambers. It has been suggested that mitogenic factor (MF) is generated by T cells only, whereas migration inhibition factor is generated by both T and B cells.

References

AGNELLO, V., WINCHESTER, R. J. and KUNKEL, H. G. (1970). *Immunology*, **19**, 909.

ALMEIDA, J. D. (1971). *Postgrad. med. J.*, **47**, 484.

ALPER, C. A. (1974). In *Structure and Function of Plasma Proteins*, Vol. 1, Chap. 7, p. 195. Ed. A. C. Allison. Plenum Press, New York and London.

BAUMAL, R. and BRODER, I. (1968). *Clin. exp. Immunol.*, **3**, 555.

BOMBARDIERI, S., LIGHTFOOT, R. W. and CHRISTIAN, C. L. (1973). *Proc. Soc. exp. Biol. Med.* **144**, 148.

CREIGHTON, D. W., LAMBERT, P. H. and MIESCHER, P. A. (1973). *J. Immunol.*, **111**, 1219.

FROLAND, S. S. and NATVIG, J. B. (1973). *Transplant. Rev.*, **16**, 114.

'IMMUNOLOGICAL METHODS': suitable reference books and manuals include:
 Handbook of Experimental Immunology, 2nd edn. (1973). Ed. D. M. Weir. Blackwell Scientific Publications, Oxford.
 Experimental Immunochemistry, 2nd ed. (1961). Ed. E. A. Kabat and M. M. Meyer. Charles C. Thomas, Springfield, Illinois.
 Cell and Tissue Culture, 4th edn. (1970). John Paul. E. and S. Livingstone, Edinburgh and London.
 In Vitro Methods in Cell-mediated Immunity. (1971). Ed. B. R. Bloom and P. R. Glade. Academic Press, New York and London.

In Vitro Methods in Cell-mediated Immunity: a progress report (1973). *Cell. Immunol.*, **6**, 331.

JOHNSON, A. H., MOWBRAY, J. F. and PORTER, K. A. (1975). *Lancet*, **1**, 762.

JONDAL, M., WIGZELL, H. and AIUTI, F. (1973). *Transplant. Rev.*, **16**, 163.

KUNKEL, H. G., MULLER-EBERHARD, H. J., FUDENBERG, H. H. and TOMASI, T. B. (1961). *J. clin. Invest.*, **40**, 117.

LACHMANN, P. J. (1975). In *Clinical Aspects of Immunology*, p. 323. Ed. P. G. H. Gell, R. R. A. Coombs and P. J. Lachmann. Blackwell Scientific Publications, Oxford.

LURHUMA, A. Z., CAMBIASO, C. L., MASSON, P. L. and HEREMANS, J. F. (1976). *Clin. exp. Immunol.* (in press).

MACLENNAN, I. (1972). *Clin. exp. Immunol.*, **10**, 275.

MELTZER, M. and FRANKLIN, E. C. (1966). *Amer. J. Med.*, **40**, 828.

NUSSENZWEIG, V. (1974). *Adv. Immunol.*, **19**, 217.

NYEDEGGER, V. E., LAMBERT, P. H., GERBER, H. and MEISCHER, P. A. (1974). *J. clin. Invest.*, **54**, 297.

ONYEWOTU, I. I., HOLBOROW, E. J. and JOHNSON, G. D. (1974). *Nature (Lond.)*, **248**, 156.

PENTTINEN, K., VAHERI, A. and MYLLYLA, G. (1971). *Clin. exp. Immunol.*, **8**, 389.

PERRIN, L. H., LAMBERT, P. H. and MIESCHER, P. A. (1975). *J. clin. Invest.*, **56**, 165.

SCHUR, P. H. and AUSTEN, E. R. F. (1971). *Bull. rheum. Dis.*, **22**, 666.

THEOFILOPOULOUS, A. N., WILSON, C. B., BOKISCH, V. A. and DIXON, F. J. (1974). *J. exp. Med.*, **140**, 1230.

WARNER, N. L. (1974). *Adv. Immunol.*, **19**, 67.

WHO/IARC—SPONSORED WORKSHOP REPORT (1974). *Scand. J. Immunol.*, **3**, 521.

WILLIAMS, B. D. and SLANEY, J. M. (1976). *Ann. rheum. Dis.* (in press).

WINCHESTER, R. J., KUNKEL, H. G. and AGNELLO, V. (1971). *J. exp. Med.*, **134**, 286 (s).

WINCHESTER, R. J., WINFIELD, J. B., SIEGAL, F., WERNET, P., BENTWICH, Z. and KUNKEL, H. G. (1974). *J. clin. Invest.*, **54**, 1082.

WINCHESTER, R. J., FU, S. M., HOFFMAN, T. and KUNKEL, H. G. (1975). *J. Immunol.*, **114**, 1210.

Section B

Applied Immunology and Connective Tissue Diseases

5

Rheumatoid Arthritis

Immunopathology of joint disease

There is a wealth of evidence which suggests that immune mechanisms participate in the pathogenesis of rheumatoid arthritis, but an assessment of their possible role requires a brief review of the clinical and pathological features of the joint disease.

The normal one- or two-cell layer thick synovial membrane and loose connective tissue, which cover the capsule of joints, become thickened in rheumatoid arthritis, and in the active phases of this chronic disease, show marked hyperaemia and exuberant villus formation. In the region of the capsular attachment to the margins of bone, where the synovium is in close approximation to the cartilaginous bone ends, characteristic erosions of cartilage and bone are found, covered with tissue, termed the pannus, which is an extension of the vascular subsynovial connective tissue and which is believed to be the source of degradative enzymes which destroy cartilage and bone, as shown in Fig. 5.1. These changes in the lining and deeper layers of synovium are accompanied by the formation of excessive amounts of synovial fluid which is made up of local secretions and blood transudate with a high protein content, a large number of polymorphs, but lesser numbers of lymphocytes, other mononuclear cells consisting of shed synovial cells as well as cells probably derived from monocytes, and secretory products of cells (e.g. immunoglobulin, lymphokines, kinins, complement, enzymes and their inhibitors). Chronic synovitis can also directly involve tendons, either because of their proximity to the joint inflammatory tissue or because of the fact that the tendons are enclosed in a fibrous sheath with a synovial lining which becomes involved by the rheumatoid process (e.g. the flexor tendons in the palms of the hands). The explanation for the loss of the remainder of the articular cartilage, which is also a feature of rheumatoid arthritis, is to some extent controversial. A thin layer of pannus extends over part of the cartilage, but other factors may include a direct degradative effect of enzymes present in the synovial fluid, accelerated mechanical wearing of cartilage that follows loss of normal joint architecture; and subchondral resorption of bone. The pressure that builds up in the diseased joint during movement may also be

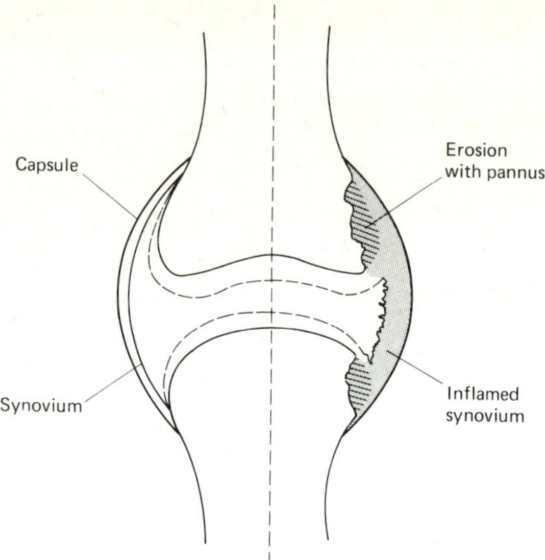

Fig. 5.1   Diagram of a joint. On the left-hand side of the dotted line is the structure of a normal joint. It shows the capsule lined with synovial membrane and, at its point of attachment to bone, its close apposition to cartilage. On the right is shown hyperplasia of inflamed synovium and erosion of cartilage and bone by pannus in rheumatoid arthritis.

responsible for the squeezing of fluid through defects into the cartilage into subchondral bone (observed as cystic erosions or 'geodes') as well as extension of the joint cavity into neighbouring soft tissues. The latter is seen particularly where a Baker's cyst communicates with the joint by a valvular mechanism or if rupture into the calf occurs. Progressive joint destruction and pain lead to loss of function and this in turn is believed to be the main factor responsible for muscle atrophy and contracture which further impair locomotor function.

These various lesions—inflammation, synovial fluid over-production, erosion of cartilage and eventual disorganization—originate from changes in the synovium which appear to be mediated by immune mechanisms. Lymphoid cells and their products (antibodies and lymphokines) engage phagocytic cells in the production and release of excessive amounts of tissue degradative enzymes from their lysosomes. There is also evidence that immune mechanisms are involved in activation of complement components (discussed below) which in turn result in the production of inflammatory and chemotactic factors. The potent inflammatory mediator, prostaglandin, has also been demonstrated in the synovial fluid and may be largely derived from the diseased synovium. A likely source is the mononuclear phagocytic cell whose activity is modulated in part by immunological stimuli.

It seems evident that there is, in addition, a regulatory defect of the immune response which may be mediated by qualitative and quantitative defects in lymphocytes or macrophages. This type of defect could result in a persistent immune response, a feature of the rheumatoid synovium also observed *in vitro* (e.g. antibody synthesis lasts for weeks under these conditions). The nature of the 'force' that drives the immune response remains elusive although it raises the question of extrinsic microbial antigens or altered autoantigens as initiating agents.

The synovium: an ectopic lymphoid organ

Microscopic examination of the rheumatoid synovial villi shows prominent number of lymphocytes, plasma cells and macrophages interspersed in a mesh-work of connective tissue (see Fig. 5.2a). The lymphocytes and plasma cells are frequently perivascular, and ultrastructural examination shows that cells belonging to both the plasma cell series and lymphoblast types are apparently in an active synthetic phase. The lining layer of the synovium is composed of two main cell types: one with the ultrastructure of phagocytes (A type) and the other with the ultrastructure of a secretory cell (B type). Both types appear to be increased in the rheumatoid synovium.

The focal chronic inflammatory reaction in the synovium has some features of a granuloma, including the formation of occasional giant cells, which are probably derived from histiocytes of macrophages. Prominent collections of lymphoid follicles are sometimes seen with pale staining cells in the central area, resembling the follicles and germinal centres of immunologically active lymph nodes. Such organization simulates changes following local antigenic challenge (see the review by Glynn, 1972). The close relationship of macrophages to lymphoblasts in the synovium has been noted by Ziff and his colleagues (Kobayashi and Ziff, 1973) who have speculated on the possibility that lymphokines produced by the lymphocytes may be exerting their activity on macrophages.

These appearances, however, did not appear to be present in the very early cases of rheumatoid arthritis reported in one series (Schumacher and Kitridou, 1972), which differed from the description of established cases in several important respects. For example, lymphocytes were only present in the perivascular areas and there was a notable absence of plasma cells, while lymphoid follicles were not observed in any of the six synovial biopsies examined (Fig. 5.2a shows such appearances). Polymorphoncnulear leucocytes were sometimes prominent in distinction to the established lesions in which they are rarely encountered. Vascular changes were also prominent and included congestion of vessels with obvious extravasation of erythrocytes whilst in venules there was evidence of a vasculitic process affecting the vessel wall characterized by polymorph and mononuclear cell infiltration.

The local synthesis of immunoglobulin is suggested by immunofluorescent studies of rheumatoid synovial membrane which show immunoglobulin within the cytoplasm of plasma cells. A minority of these Ig-producing cells stain for rheumatoid factor (anti-Ig) activity (Mellors et al., 1961). Other studies have suggested that rheumatoid factor is blocked by IgG and represents a large proportion of the immunoglobulin synthesized and is only revealed after pepsin digestion (Natvig et al., 1975). It has been demonstrated that the rheumatoid synovium is capable of synthesizing immunoglobulin in quantities similar to that produced by lymph nodes or splenic tissue in culture (Smiley et al., 1968).

(a)

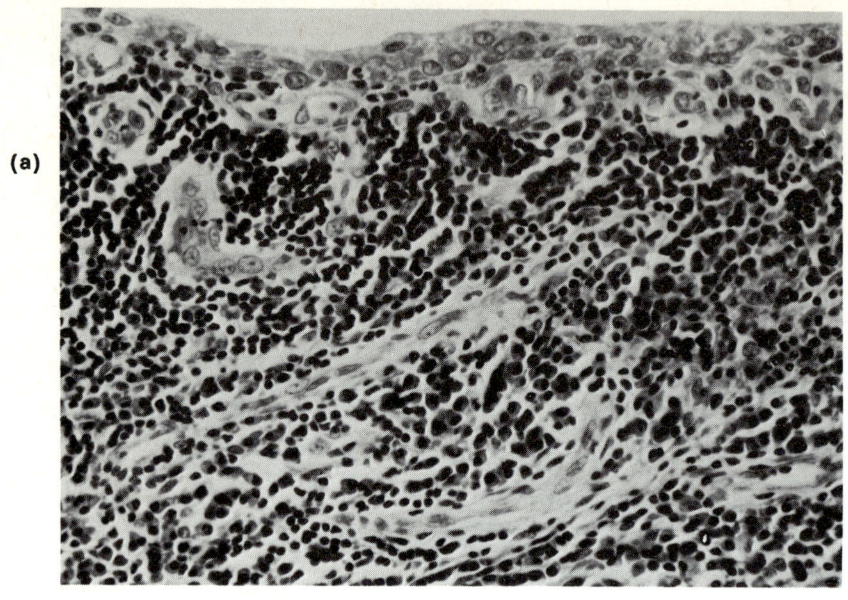

(b)

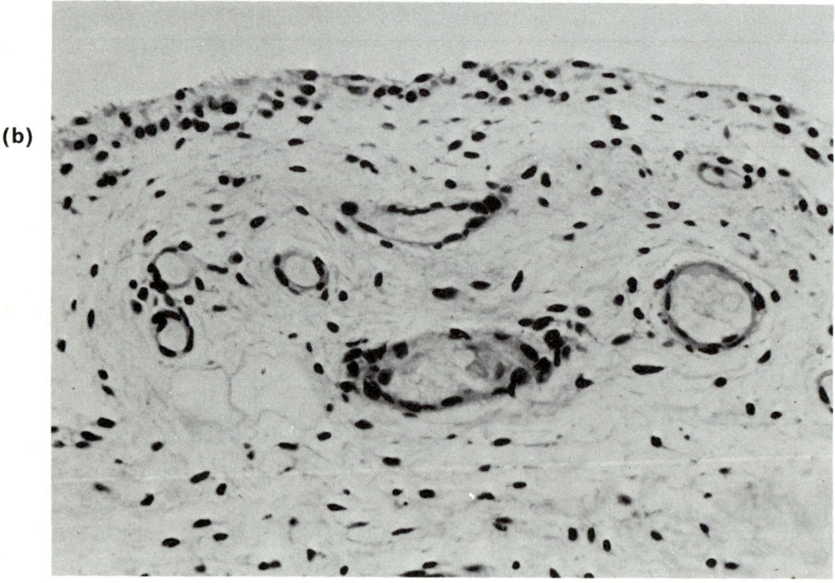

Fig. 5.2 Two types of rheumatoid synovial tissue, showing: (**a**) hyperplasia of the lining layer with subsynovial mononuclear (lymphocyte, plasma cell and macrophage) infiltration and dilatation of blood vessels; (**b**) dilated subsynovial blood vessels with some perivascular mononuclear cells.

Experiments with synovial explant cultures have also demonstrated their capacity to produce lymphokines with MIF and mitogenic factor activity (Stastny *et al.*, 1975). The ability of the rheumatoid synovium to function as an ectopic lymphoid organ capable of intense local immunological reactivity is probably relevant to the role that it plays in perpetuating chronic inflammation and causing damage to the joint.

In addition to synovial production of immunoglobulin and lymphokines, it is likely that its macrophages also synthesize complement components, and recent evidence implicates the synovium in local production of prostaglandins as well as lysosomal enzymes and possibly protease inhibitors (see Table 5.1), thus providing evidence of a functionally independent organ.

Table 5.1 Synthesis of biologically active molecules by the synovium in rheumatoid arthritis

Product	Cell involved
Antibody	Plasma cells
Lymphokines	T cells
Complement	? Macrophages
Prostaglandins	? Macrophages
Lysosomal hydrolases	Lining cells (A type)
	Macrophages
? Trypsin inhibitors α1 and α2	? Lining cells (B type)

Immune complexes in synovial membrane and fluid

Examination of rheumatoid synovial membrane by immunofluorescent techniques has shown IgG and complement components (usually together) or IgG and IgM as large or smaller whispy deposits in the interstitium of the membrane (reviewed by Zvaifler, 1973). In sero-positive patients IgM has been detected in the synovium, usually in the absence of complement component C3 (Fish *et al.*, 1966). Isolated lining cells obtained by trypsin digestion of biopsy samples have shown phagocytosed immunofluorescent material, the typical combination being IgG and C3 or IgG and anti-IgG (rheumatoid factor) (Kinsella *et al.*, 1970). These studies therefore suggest that immune complexes consisting of rheumatoid factor bound to its antigen (immunoglobulin) and binding complement are not uncommon in the synovial membrane although their amount is controversial. The precise nature of the antigen to which the rest of the IgG is bound remains unknown.

Elution studies have demonstrated IgG–anti–IgG complexes (the anti-IgG being rheumatoid factors of IgG and IgM class) as well as complexes of Fab fragments and antibody. It seems likely that the immune reactants which form the complexes are all produced locally. The possibility has been considered that the synovial cells may themselves be a source of antigens, either in their naturally occurring or in a modified form, possibly as a result of infection (Chapter 3).

Evidence for the presence of immune complexes in synovial fluid is very strong. A factor resembling soluble antigen–antibody complexes has been reported in three-quarters of rheumatoid synovial fluid examined by the measurement of histamine release from guinea-pig lungs (Baumal and Broder, 1968). The direct demonstration of immune complexes in synovial fluids by the use of ultra-centrifugation was reported by Kunkel and his associates (1961) who have subsequently shown that the complexes are mainly composed of IgG associated with rheumatoid factor. Using precipitation methods Winchester *et al.* (1971) from the same laboratory have shown that the majority of rheumatoid joint fluids contain a high molecular weight complex, which reacts with C1q or rheumatoid factor. Elution of the complex from its reactant, C1q or rheumatoid factor, showed that it comprised easily dissociable IgG–anti-IgG, thus suggesting that the predominant complex in synovial fluid is that made up by immunoglobulin linked to IgG rheumatoid factor. Hannestad (1967) has reported material resembling aggregated IgG in synovial fluids which dissociates at low pH and consists partly of IgM rheumatoid factor. Cryoprecipitates containing IgG, IgM rheumatoid factors, C1q, DNA and anti-nuclear antibodies have been detected in synovial fluids from rheumatoid patients and indicate further the presence of immune complexes. Rheumatoid joint fluids also frequently contain antibodies to nuclei of granulocyte polymorphs, and since a large number of granulocytes may be constantly breaking down in the fluid releasing their nuclear antigens, yet another type of immune complex is probably being generated. These complexes could undoubtedly serve to perpetuate the chronic inflammatory reaction present in rheumatoid joints.

The finding of immune complexes within the leucocytes of synovial fluid (Hurd *et al.*, 1970) and phagocytic cells of the synovial membrane provides a basis for the view that phagocytosis of complexes may be the important activity which leads to the generation of increased amounts of lysosomal enzymes with tissue degrading activity. It was of interest to note that whereas polymorphs (from any source) incubated with joint fluids of sero-positive patients readily phagocytose complexes, incubation with joint fluids of sero-negative patients (also containing complexes) only develop intracellular inclusions of complexes if IgM rheumatoid factor is added. Thus IgM rheumatoid factor appears to alter soluble complexes in a manner which encourages phagocytosis.

Circulating immune complexes and vasculitis

By using analytical ultracentrifugation, Kunkel and his colleagues (1961) showed the presence of immune complexes which sedimented between 7 and 19S as well as 19S IgM complexed to 7S producing a 22S band in the serum of patients with rheumatoid arthritis. Winchester *et al.* (1971) have investigated this phenomenon further using monoclonal and polyclonal IgM rheumatoid factors and C1q for precipitation of immune complexes present in rheumatoid sera. Only complexes precipitated with monoclonal rheumatoid factor were detected in the sera of rheumatoid patients, whereas joint fluids gave reactions with C1q and polyclonal rheumatoid factor as well, suggesting dissimilarities in the composition of the complex in blood and synovial fluid. It was further noted that the immune complexes in rheumatoid sera did not fix C1q (whereas synovial fluid complexes did) and this was in keeping with the observed changes in complement in rheumatoid arthritis. However, more sensitive techniques have recently shown C1q binding by the majority of rheumatoid sera (Lambert *et al*, 1975), indicating that the differences between blood and synovial fluid are probably quantitative.

Although the role of circulating immune complexes in rheumatoid arthritis is not clear, their involvement in the genesis of severe disease and vasculitis is supported by a number of observations. In a study reported by Weisman and Zvaifler (1975) cryoprecipitates containing IgG, IgM, C3 and anti-nuclear factors occurred in the sera of rheumatoid patients with the most severe disease, and the highest levels were observed when vasculitis was also evident. Complement consumption, presumably instituted by immune complexes, was presumed to occur from the inverse correlation of C3 levels with the amount of cryoglobulins. An increased catabolic rate of complement component C3 in patients with vasculitis has been documented and suggests immune complex fixation and consumption (Weinstein *et al.*, 1972), although other workers have found this to be the case even in patients whose disease is confined to joints. Although Douglas (1965) failed to demonstrate IgM rheumatoid factor in the bland intimal lesions of digital vessels from rheumatoid patients, IgG, IgM and C3 have been demonstrated in an actively inflamed blood vessel supplying the sural nerve of a patient with neuropathy due to rheumatoid vasculitis, whilst an endarteritis compatible with the healing stage of a similar process was suspected in four other biopsies (Conn *et al.*, 1972). However, it is important to note that circulating complexes in vasculitis complicating rheumatoid arthritis, for reasons not well understood, are of a type that do not appear to be nephritogenic.

A recent report has drawn attention to the possibility that leucopenia in patients with Felty's syndrome (lymphadenopathy, splenomegaly associated with anaemia, leucopenia and thrombocytopenia) is associated with depressed leucocyte function resulting from ingestion of circulating immune complexes.

Nodules

Patients with appreciable quantities of IgM rheumatoid factor frequently develop nodules in subcutaneous tissues characterized by a central area of necrosis and a surrounding pallisade of epithelioid cells with variable degrees of lymphocyte and plasma cell infiltration and vasculitis. The presence of immunoglobulin (including rheumatoid factor) and complement in the necrotic areas has been demonstrated but may have little pathogenetic significance in such a situation. On the other hand, antibody synthesis in the nodule may indicate an active local immune process which may well be relevant to pathogenetic mechanisms. Environmental factors (movement and trauma) also play an eventual part in nodule production, as they may indeed do in the development of rheumatoid synovitis itself. These patients are also liable to develop multi-system involvement; for example, the protean manifestations of vasculitis, serositis and fibrosing alveolitis.

Complement

Synovial fluid complement levels measured by the functional haemolytic assay have been found to be lower in rheumatoid synovitis than patients with osteoarthrosis (reviewed by Schur and Austen, 1971 and Zvaifler, 1973). The reduced haemolytic complement level shows a relationship to the presence of rheumatoid factor in serum and in the fluid itself. The early components C4 and C2 are lowered in synovial fluid, suggesting that immune complex activation of complement is usually operative. However, it should be noted that where evidence of the alternate pathway has been sought by investigating levels of properdin or complement proactivator (factor B) in synovial fluids, it appears that this too is being utilized (Ruddy *et al.*, 1975). There is the additional possibility that plasmin and proteases, present in the synovial fluid, may also directly activate various complement components.

Activation of complement leads to the generation of a variety of biological activities which are relevant to the rheumatoid process, in particular the attraction of a large number of polymorphs, estimated to be in the region of a few billion cells every 24 hours; increased vascular permeability; enhanced phagocytosis; and co-operation with cellular immune mechanisms. Synovial fluid complement levels in very early cases of rheumatoid arthritis also usually show evidence of consumption, thus raising the possibility that complement contributes to the perpetuation of the chronic inflammatory process from an early stage of the disease.

In the synovial membrane, deposition of the C3 component of complement has been regularly shown in association with IgG, both in the form of extracellular, interstitial deposits and as phagocytosed material in the A type phagocytic lining cells. The presumption is that complement is attached to immune complexes; the nature of the antigen, however, is not always known although it has been pointed out that IgG itself may be the immunogen.

Studies of complement components in the blood of patients with 'uncomplicated' rheumatoid arthritis do not usually show reduced levels either of total activity or of individual components, and may indeed show a rise. But consistently slightly lowered levels occur in sero-positive patients when compared with other forms of inflammatory arthritis in which complement levels are often elevated. Since blood levels of complement are the result of a dynamic equilibrium between synthesis and utilization or normal catabolism, the increased synthesis which appears to occur during an inflammatory process may effectively mask the true extent of its utilization. Studies with radio-labelled complement C3, which measure the turnover of the labelled material in the circulation, however, do show an increased breakdown or consumption of C3 especially in sero-positive patients. Another approach to the study of turnover of complement is related to the observation that activation of complement is accompanied by the generation of stable inactivation products derived from C3 and C4 (and termed C3i and C4i). These have been found in the synovial fluid and sera of patients with rheumatoid arthritis (Versey *et al.*, 1973). In a study of C3i and C4i in blood, the levels of the two products changed together, indicating participation of the early complement pathway. It is of interest that no evidence of decreased synthesis of complement in rheumatoid arthritis has been described, unlike some cases of SLE.

Rheumatoid factors

Agglutination tests for IgM rheumatoid factor, such as the sheep cell agglutination of Rose–Waaler (Rose *et al.*, 1948) and the latex agglutination test employing latex particles coated with F-11 fraction of IgG (Singer, 1961), are positive in 60–70 per cent of patients with rheumatoid arthritis. There is a large variation in titre, not only between different patients, but often in the same patient on sequential sampling and different stages of the disease: titres do not necessarily reflect the disease activity accurately. The appearance of rheumatoid factors can precede clinical signs of disease or occur subsequently. The presence of rheumatoid factor is however associated with a poor over-all prognosis and together with the presence of nodules is almost invariably present when vasculitis supervenes. Detailed studies have shown that the joint lesions are worse in sero-positive patients than those who are sero-negative.

As previously discussed (Chapter 3), rheumatoid factors have been implicated as an important component of immune complexes in the synovial fluid of rheumatoid arthritis, and it has been suggested that both IgG and IgM classes of rheumatoid factor are involved in activation of complement, enhanced phagocytosis and consequent increased production and release of lysosomal enzymes. The results from a series of studies in which IgG or its fragments were injected into the knee joints of rheumatoid and control subjects indicate that acute inflammatory reactions occur under circumstances in which complex formation with rheumatoid factors might take place (Rawson *et al.*, 1970). In these experiments the most severe inflammatory changes were observed when autologous IgG or Fc fragments were used, suggesting the autoimmune nature of the response.

From the point of view of its detection as an aid to diagnosis in rheumatic diseases it is generally agreed that the sheep cell agglutination test of Rose–Waaler, when positive in a titre of 1–32 or more, has a high degree of specificity for rheumatoid arthritis; the latex agglutination test, although more sensitive, is less diagnostically specific. In practice, both tests should be used together to provide complementary information. The multiplicity of test systems and the general lack of use of standardized methods, however, lead to problems of interpretation and it is to be hoped that international standardization promoted by WHO receives wider support.

Relative importance of humoral and cellular immunity in pathogenesis

The relative importance of antibody-mediated or lymphocyte-mediated immunity in the pathogenesis of rheumatoid arthritis remains a subject of current investigation (see Chapter 2). The observation that hypogammaglobulinaemic children develop a syndrome resembling rheumatoid arthritis has been put forward as evidence that cellular mechanisms are of greater importance in the rheumatoid synovitis process. Further evidence for this belief centres around the histological observations mentioned already, and from the study of experimental models of arthritis, in which cellular mechanisms are capable of transferring synovitis from one animal to another. Experiments in the chicken in which bursectomy or thymectomy can lead to the biological separation of cellular- and antibody-mediated mechanisms have shown that an immune synovitis may be produced in the absence of the thymus or bursa, but that the full evolution of the granulomatous type lesion in the synovium required both systems. Thus it is likely that both the cellular and the humoral mechanisms are acting in concert but that each, in its own right, may be able to produce synovitis.

Lymphocytes in synovial membrane and fluid

Attempts at classifying the type of lymphocyte in rheumatoid synovium have been made by a study of the inter-relationship of lymphocytes with cells whose ultrastructure is compatible with that of plasma cells or lymphoblasts, within the subsynovial infiltrate, and it was concluded that B cells predominate although T cells are also present (Kobayashi and Ziff, 1973). These indirect observations are open to different interpretations and the presently used more direct methods employing E, EA and EAC rosette formation or immunofluorescent methods on frozen tissue sections are insufficiently studied to draw any firm conclusions. In a study on fresh tissue sections of synovial membrane some lymphocytes in the germinal centres and lymphoid aggregates showed rosette formation with EAC cells (a marker of B cells); the remaining majority showed no reaction with EAC or sheep erythrocytes (a marker of T cells) (Tannenbaum *et al.*, 1975). A preponderance of E-rosette-forming (T) cells, was however, observed in another study in which lymphocyte suspensions from synovial membrane were obtained following digestion with collagenase and deoxyribonuclease (Van Boxel and Paget, 1975).

A number of studies on the composition of lymphocyte subpopulations in synovial fluid have been reported with variable results. An increased percentage of EAC and surface Ig positive cells (B lymphocytes) was noted compared to blood in one study, whilst the findings of a similar number of surface Ig-positive cells in synovial fluid and peripheral blood was reported in another study, reduced numbers being found in others. Using fluoresceinated aggregated IgG as a marker for B cells, a lower percentage figure was also found in synovial fluid compared with blood. An increased proportion of synovial fluid lymphocytes form E-rosettes compared with blood lymphocytes (Winchester *et al.*, 1973; Sheldon *et al.*, 1974). However, the studies are difficult to assess since the proportion of cells which were claimed to belong to one population or another varied, presumably due to technical reasons. Moreover, absolute numbers were not usually available, and clinical details are lacking, so that strict comparison between studies are difficult to make.

Lymphocyte subpopulations in peripheral blood

Several studies on lymphocyte subpopulations in peripheral blood and synovial fluid have been published with conflicting results and conclusions. Using the technique of sheep cell rosette formation, the percentage of lymphocytes characterized as T cells by different investigators in control subjects and patients with rheumatoid arthritis have varied enormously; for example, in one study (Keith and Currey, 1973) the proportion of T cells in rheumatoid patients was estimated to be approximately 30 per cent, whereas in another (Winchester *et al.*, 1973) they constituted up to 92 per cent of the total lymphocyte population. In the former study it was claimed that the percentage of T cells estimated in rheumatoid subjects was higher than in controls, but several other groups, whilst estimating a different percentage figure of T cells, agree with the conclusion of Winchester and his colleagues that similar values are obtained in patients with rheumatoid arthritis and controls. Using fluoresceinated anti-T cell antiserum for detection of T cells, Williams and his colleagues (1973) have estimated that one-third of their rheumatoid patients, including several with active arthritis, had a proportion of T cells less than the lowest figure of 40 per cent observed in controls (mean 75 per cent); and in RA patients whose disease was quiescent or relatively less active, the numbers of T cells were higher.

Estimation of circulating B cells has likewise yielded different percentage figures even when apparently similar techniques have been used. In a study using $F(ab^1)_2$ fragments of anti-Ig sera a mean of about 6 per cent lymphocytes were positive for the main classes of surface Ig (most commonly staining simultaneously for both IgD and IgM), and no significant differences between RA patients and controls were observed (Winchester *et al.*, 1975).

Bach and his colleagues (1970) reported a population of circulating lymphocytes in peripheral blood which formed rosettes with human erythrocytes sensitized with rabbit IgG antibody found in increased numbers in rheumatoid arthritis. This was termed the 'rheumatoid rosette' (RR). These French investigators have documented in large surveys that 75–80 per cent of patients with rheumatoid arthritis possess more than 6/1,000 RR-forming lymphocytes, whereas 90–95 per cent of normal subjects have less than this number in their peripheral blood. This increased number was observed irrespective of whether the patients were sero-positive or sero-negative for IgM rheumatoid factor tests. An inexplicably high incidence of RR occurred in patients with gout, degenerative arthritis and other less well defined rheumatic syndromes. It has been suggested that the sensitized erythrocytes binding with lymphocytes are a cellular analogue of the reaction between sensitized red cells and rheumatoid factor anti-globulins as observed in agglutination tests (for example the Rose–Waaler or latex tests). However, the sensitized erythrocyte used in the RR test might also be expected to form EA rosettes with Fc-receptor-bearing lymphocytes present on different subpopulations; e.g. Ig-positive B cells and K cells. Recent investigations (J. Sany, personal communication) suggest that the RR-forming lymphocyte is in all probability a Fc-receptor-bearing lymphocyte which is Ig- and E-negative, and has a high avidity for human red cell sensitized with rabbit antibody under the conditions used for performing the test, which include a short incubation period. This explanation, together with the other peculiarities of different EA systems discussed under methodological considerations (Chapter 4), may account for the fact that other investigators have failed to substantiate any difference between RA patients and controls.

In a number of studies in which enumeration of B and T cells has been undertaken it was noted that the total did not reach 100 per cent. The unlabelled cells have been termed 'null' cells, a concept which, in view of the foregoing comments of methodology, will be noted as being rather nebulous and speculative. However, emphasis has been laid on the increased number of 'null' cells in RA patients compared with controls, especially in active disease.

Immune status

The immune status of patients with rheumatoid arthritis has been extensively investigated, but in this field also there does not seem to be general agreement about the findings either in relation to delayed hypersensitivity or to the humoral immune response. The results obtained in various studies, the reasons for possible reported differences and their possible clinical significance are reviewed below.

Impairment of cell-mediated immune responses in patients with rheumatoid arthritis has been suggested by various observations, although the degree and frequency of impairment remain controversial owing to lack of confirmation of the claims in independent laboratories. These difficulties arise partly from problems of standardization of the large number of different tests used, their interpretation in terms of whether they test T or B cell function, and the effect of drugs, and poor general health. Furthermore, since the mechanism of particular lymphocyte function tests remains uncertain, it has not been possible to differentiate clearly between functional defects and depressed function arising as a result of a change in the number of T cells, a defect in helper effects of macrophages, and the interfering effects of serum factors (e.g. immune complexes and lymphocyte autoantibodies). An impaired capacity to induce contact-type hypersensitivity to dinitrochlorobenzene (DNCB) has been described in some patients with RA (Leventhal *et al.*, 1967; Whaley *et al.*, 1971). Delayed hypersensitivity tests with antigens (e.g. tuberculin PPD, mumps antigen and brucellin) have been reported to be depressed, but in one study were related to the degree of functional disability and poor general health (Hayes *et al.*, 1970) and in another study were observed only in patients who also had features of Sjögren's syndrome (Whaley *et al.*, 1971). In another study (Houba *et al.*, 1964) smaller reactions to streptococcal antigens were noted in RA patients compared with osteoarthrosis. Our own experience suggests that skin tests to antigens may indeed be depressed but patients are rarely anergic and frequently respond to one or another antigen if a battery of tests is employed. In some patients subjected to repeated testing, the reactions were boosted (Maini *et al.*, 1976).

Lymphocyte transformation *in vitro* with common antigens, unless absent (which is rare), can only be interpreted in relation to control groups which are difficult to define, and, when observed, such a finding may not be specific for rheumatoid arthritis since it is common in a variety of chronic diseases. One-way mixed leucocyte reactions (MLR) using stimulator cells derived from healthy donors have been reported to be occasionally absent or normal. When rheumatoid lymphocytes are used as stimulator cells there is more general agreement that MLR is depressed or absent, although this may be due to the fact that certain genetically controlled lymphocyte surface alloantigens are shared by patients with rheumatoid arthritis and consequently do not stimulate the responder cells (Chapter 13). Responses to PHA have been reported to be depressed, or to show borderline depression, and there is evidence of abnormal dose-response curves with both hypo- and hyper-reactive populations (reviewed by Tannenbaum and Schur, 1974). Pokeweed mitogen (PWM) responses have been reported to be normal (indicating normal B cell response). In another study lymphocyte binding of radioiodine-labelled PHA and concanavalin A were studied, and the former only was reported to be below the binding level of control lymphocytes (Rawson and Huang, 1974).

In a study of the spontaneous 'background' uptake of ^{3}H-thymidine within a few hours of venesection, leucocytes from rheumatoid patients have been reported to show an increased level compared to normal, a finding which might suggest the possibility of a carry-over of a high *in vivo* stimulation of lymphocytes due to a hyperimmune state, although activated monocytes may contribute to this phenomenon (Horwitz *et al.*, 1970).

Synovial fluid lymphocyte transformation reactions have been compared with studies on peripheral blood and reported to show depressed reactions to PHA (Sheldon *et al.*, 1974). In another study, lymphocyte transformation by antigen of synovial fluid lymphocytes was depressed compared with peripheral blood lymphocyte reactions, but a greater stimulation with lipopolysaccharide (LPS) was noted, the results suggesting B cell functional over-activity, and T cell hyporeactivity (Ivanyi *et al.*, 1973). Maclennan and Loewi (1970) measured lymphocyte-mediated cytotoxicity on allogeneic target cells and showed an increased activity using rheumatoid synovial fluid lymphocytes compared with lymphocytes obtained from the blood of the patients (the latter showing the same activity as lymphocytes from normal controls). It is possible to suggest that the T-enriched synovial fluid lymphocyte population is poorly responsive to PHA and antigens due to stimulation *in vivo*, and prior 'commitment'; the increased cytotoxicity of these cells could also be accounted for on this basis.

It is extremely probable that lymphocytes have an effector role in the rheumatoid joint. Evidence for the presence of B cells, T cells or K cells is directly (or indirectly) obtainable in rheumatoid synovial membrane or synovial fluid. The possibility that they are involved in the inflammatory process in the synovium joint is further supported by the observation that complement levels in synovial fluid are most depressed when the lymphocyte infiltration is marked and that active villus formation observed at arthroscopy was associated with heavy lymphocyte infiltration (Yates and Scott, 1975). The possibility that heavy lymphocyte infiltration ultimately correlates with less severe cartilage destruction has also been put forward (Muirden and Mills, 1971). This is not necessarily inconsistent with the other observations since it could be argued that the lymphocyte-rich synovitis, although associated with severe inflammatory changes, is also likely to limit the initiating stimulus. Thus there may be a basis for the clinical observation that an acute onset of inflammatory arthritis may have a good prognosis, whereas recurrently active disease, often with an insidious onset, ends in joint destruction.

The ability of rheumatoid arthritis patients to form antibodies on stimulation with antigens has been investigated by a number of workers. Both primary responses utilizing microbial antigens such as flagellin and Brucella (which most individuals have not previously come across), as well as secondary immune responses, employing tetanus or diphtheria antigen (with which the majority have previously been immunized), have been used in these studies. The results have varied; the responses have been: the same as control groups, higher than control groups, or depressed compared with control groups. These discrepancies have probably arisen from the selection of patients or controls as well as the lack of standardization of the antigen employed. The studies are therefore inconclusive, but it can be said that none of them has really demonstrated any significant abnormality in the quantity of antibody generated by the rheumatoid individual.

The possibility that antibody deficiency may be involved in the pathology of rheumatoid arthritis has been suggested by the description of a rheumatoid-like syndrome in a significant number of children with hypogammaglobulinaemia. However, essential differences from rheumatoid arthritis remain, including the lack of an erosive arthritis. Arthritis of this type responds to treatment with immunoglobulin and does not seem to occur (in the first place) if the children have been treated with adequate replacement doses of immunoglobulin. IgA deficiency in rheumatoid arthritis patients has also been described as occurring more frequently than might be expected by chance. It is possible, therefore, that selective or total immunoglobulin deficiency may be one predisposing factor in a multifactorial disease such as rheumatoid arthritis.

The importance of additional serum factors which could modify the immune response has been characterized by the finding of anti-lymphocyte antibodies (cytotoxin) in sera of patients with rheumatoid arthritis (Williams *et al.*, 1971). Such cytotoxins may underlie the possible loss of reactivity being measured by the various tests, and, more importantly, also indicate a possible mechanism for loss of T cell tolerance or suppressor cell activity (Chapter 13).

Immune status in juvenile rheumatoid arthritis (JRA)

Delayed hypersensitivity reactions to antigen preparations of Candida, streptokinase-streptodornase (SKSD), mumps, Brucella and tubercluin PPD were measured in JRA patients and in age- and sex-matched controls (Hoyeral, 1973). In this study, patients' reactions to these antigens were less than in controls, but the differences to individual antigens reached statistical significance only for Brucella and mumps virus. An over-all score for delayed hypersensitivity was calculated by adding the diameter of induration to all antigens tested, and this was also found to be significantly less in JRA than in controls, the difference being most striking in male patients. On this basis it has been suggested that cellular hypersensitivity in JRA is depressed. In a study in which reactions to antigen preparations of Candida and SKSD were studied simultaneously using skin tests, lymphocyte transformation tests and migration inhibition factor (MIF) production, a number of children were encountered in whom, in spite of negative skin tests, lymphocyte transformation and/or MIF were positive (Panush *et al.*, 1972). The finding of a dissociation between *in vivo* and *in vitro* tests has been noted in other chronic diseases, including SLE (Horwitz, 1972), but its significance is not fully understood.

Immune reactions to infective agents

The possibility that rheumatoid arthritis is due to an infection remains an attractive hypothesis because it would readily explain the clinical, pathological and serological features of the disease. The clinical features such as weight loss, fever, anaemia, leucocytosis, a polymorph-rich synovial fluid and a raised ESR, suggest chronic infection, whilst the synovial pathology is compatible with a process intiated and perpetuated by a persistent infection with attendant release of mircobial antigens and associated antimicrobial and autoallergic immune responses.

Improved methods for culturing organisms such as mycoplasmas and viruses, as well as a better understanding of the biology of viruses, especially in relation to their role in oncogenesis and slow virus infection, have lead to a renewed search for such agents. Similarly, there has been better understanding of the immune processes involved in infections. We must consider the possibility, not only that rheumatoid arthritis may be caused by an unusual organism and an immune response directed towards this, but also that the disease may result from an abnormal host immune response to common microbial agents. The possible role of viruses in rheumatoid arthritis has been reviewed by Hamerman (1975).

Virus isolation studies have so far been uniformly unsuccessful in rheumatoid arthritis. Electron microscopic observations of endothelial inclusions resembling viruses have been reported by Neumark and Farkas (1970) but have not been confirmed in other laboratories. Surveys of antibody responses to well recognized viruses such as measles, herpes simplex, mumps, adenovirus and para-influenza have yielded no consistent results. There is a suggestion that the measles antibody is marginally raised, although not as obviously as in SLE; rubella antibodies may also be raised. The titre of antibodies to herpes simplex, on the other hand, is reported to be lower than expected in rheumatoid patients, as was the lymphocyte transformation response. It has been pointed out that this latter observation may only reflect the interference by rheumatoid factor in the detection of antibodies to herpes simplex and, when this is absorbed out, levels to the virus are in fact higher than in controls.

Indirect evidence for virus infection was obtained by the study of Grayzel and Beck (1970) who found that rheumatoid synovial cells in culture were unduly resistant to deliberate infection *in vitro* by rubella virus. Furthermore, they found that this resistance could be induced in rabbit synovium by injection of rabbit joints with rheumatoid synovial cells, as well as by cell fusion between cultured rabbit and human rheumatoid synovial cells. The lack of success with deliberate infection of cultured cells was interpreted as indicating interference due to pre-existing virus infection in the cell, and furthermore its transmission *in vivo* and *in vitro* was put forward as supporting the idea of a transmissible agent. However, the inability to infect rheumatoid culture cells may result from the production of a shell of hyaluronic acid which is impenetrable by virus, since treatment of cells to remove hyaluronic acid was followed by ability to infect them with vesicular stomatitis virus (Patterson *et al.*, 1973). Further, other laboratories have been unable to confirm the observation that rheumatoid cells are less susceptible to *in vitro* viral infection and the results remain controversial.

Recent evidence put forward that rubella specific antigens are coded on the surface of rheumatoid synovial fibroblasts, as detected by a cytotoxic assay using primate anti-rubella antibody (Patterson *et al.*, 1973), has again raised the possibility that rubella virus may be of aetiological significance in rheumatoid arthritis. If this were indeed the case, it might be predicted that rheumatoid arthritis would follow outbreaks of rubella or following immunization. In fact, although a polyarthritis resembling rheumatoid does occur in a significant number of individuals who have suffered from rubella or who have been vaccinated, there are important distinguishing features. The disease is always self-limiting, and the synovial fluid contains large mononuclear cells in sharp contrast to the largely polymorph exudate of rheumatoid arthritis. There is only one recorded case which seemingly progressed to classical rheumatoid arthritis.

The report that *Mycoplasma fermentans* could be isolated in up to 40 per cent of synovial fluid in rheumatoid arthritis acquired special significance when it was also found that cell-mediated immunity to its antigens was demonstrable in only rheumatoid patients (Williams *et al.*, 1970). The possibility that the cell-mediated immunity to *Mycoplasma fermentans* may in fact be demonstrable in the leucocyte migration test, because of the contaminating IgG in the Mycoplasma preparation, was investigated further by using Mycoplasma cultured in media free of immunoglobulin. Such antigens, whilst possessing specific determinants of Mycoplasma, were found to show virtually no inhibition compared with Mycoplasma antigens prepared in serum rich in immunoglobulin (Maini *et al.*, 1975). However, the fact that the cellular immunity in rheumatoid patients may be directed to IgG, possibly also by its attachment to Mycoplasma membrane, still appears an attractive hypothesis, provided the organisms can be isolated from rheumatoid arthritis patients; but several recent studies have failed to isolate the organism.

The isolation of diphtheroid-like organisms from synovial fluid has been claimed by workers from Professor Duthie's laboratories in Edinburgh. These observations have been confirmed in another laboratory which has also reported the finding of specific corynebacterial antigens and antibody in rheumatoid synovial fluid. Such organisms, however, are frequently found as commensals, and they may infect rheumatoid joints secondarily. Their main biological significance may lie in the fact that they are powerful adjuvants (Stewart *et al.*, 1969).

References

BACH, J. F., DELRIEU, F. and DELBARRE, F. (1970). *Amer. J. Med.*, **49**, 213.

BAUMAL, R. and BRODER, I. (1968). *Clin. exp. Immunol.*, **3**, 555.

CONN, D. L., MCDUFFIE, F. C. and DYCK, P. J. (1972). *Arthr. and Rheum.*, **15**, 135.

DOUGLAS, W. (1965). *Ann. rheum. Dis.*, **24**, 40.

FISH, A. J., MICHAEL, A. F., GERWUTZ, H. and GOOD, R. A. (1966). *Arthr. and Rheum.*, **9**, 267.

GLYNN, L. E. (1972). *Ann. rheum. Dis.*, **31**, 412.

GRAYZEL, A. I. and BECK, C. (1970). *J. exp. Med.*, **131**, 367.

HAMERMAN, D. (1975). In *Immunological Basis of Connective Tissue Disorders*, p. 17. Ed. L. G. Silvestri. North Holland Publishing Co., Amsterdam.

HANNESTAD, K. (1967). *Clin. exp. Immunol.*, **2**, 511.

HAYES, J. R., WARD, D. J. and JENNINGS, J. F. (1970). In *Impaired Cell-mediated Hypersensitivity in Man*, p. 37. Ed. J. F. Jennings and D. J. Ward. Orthopaedic Hospital, Oswestry, England.

HORWITZ, D. A., STASTNY, P. and ZIFF, M. (1970). *J. Lab. clin. Med.*, **76**, 391.

HOUBA, V., ADAM, M., MALECEK, J. and TEASSERK, B. (1964). *Experimentia*, **20**, 522.

HOYERAL, H. M. (1973). *Ann. rheum. Dis.*, **32**, 331.

HURD, E. R., LOSPALLUTO, J. and ZIFF, M. (1970). *Arthr. and Rheum.*, **13**, 724.

IVANYI, L., LEHNER, T. and BURRY, H. C. (1973). *Immunology*, **25**, 905.

KEITH, H. I. and CURREY, H. L. F. (1973). *Ann. rheum. Dis.*, **32**, 202.

KINSELLA, T. D., BAUM, J. and ZIFF, M. (1970). *Arthr. and Rheum.*, **13**, 734.

KOBAYASHI, I. and ZIFF, M. (1973). *Arthr. and Rheum.*, **16**, 471.

KUNKEL, H. G., MULLER-EBERHARD, H. J., FUDENBERG, H. H. and TOMASI, T. B. (1961). *J. clin. Invest.*, **40**, 117.

LAMBERT, P. H., NYEDEGGER, U. E., PERRIN, L. H., MCCORMICK, J., FEHR, K. and MIESCHER, P. (1975). *Rheumatology*, **6**, 52.

LEVENTHAL, B. G., WALDORF, D. S. and TALAL, N. (1967). *J. clin. Invest.*, **46**, 1338.

MACLENNAN, I. C. M. and LOEWI, G. (1970). *Clin. exp. Immunol.*, **6**, 713.

MAINI, R. N., LEMCKE, R. M., WINDSOR, G. D., ROFFE, L.M., MAGRATH, I. T. and DUMONDE, D. C. (1975). *Rheumatology*, **5**, 118.

MAINI, R. N., SCOTT, J. T., ROFFE, L., HAMBLIN, A. and DUMONDE, D. C. (1976). In *Infection and Immunity*, p. 579. Ed. D. C. Dumonde. Blackwell Scientific Publications, Oxford.

MELLORS, R. C., NOWOSLAWSKI, A. and KORNGOLD, L. (1961). *Amer J. Path.*, **39**, 533.

MUIRDEN, K. D. and MILLS, K. W. (1971). *Brit. med. J.*, **4**, 219.

NATVIG, J. B., MUNTHE, E. and PAHLE, J. (1975). *Rheumatology*, **6**, 167.

NEUMARK, T. and FARKAS, K. (1970). *Ann. rheum. Dis.*, **29**, 653.

PANUSH, R. S., BIANCO, N. E., SCHUR, P. H., ROCKLIN, R. E., DAVID, J. R. and STILLMAN, J. S. (1972). *Clin. exp. Immunol.*, **10**, 103.

PATTERSON, R., HOWARD, R. and DEINHARDT, F. (1973). *Clin. Res.*, **28**, 878.

RAWSON, A. J. and HUANG, T. C. (1974). *Clin. exp. Immunol.*, **16**, 47.

RAWSON, A. J., HOLLANDER, J. L., QUISMORIO, F. P. and ABELSON, N. M. (1970). In *Immune Complex Diseases*, p. 69. Ed. L. Bonomo and J. L. Turk. Carlo Erba Foundation, Milan.

ROSE, H. E., RAGAN, C., PEARCE, E. and LIPMAN, M. O. (1948). *Proc. Soc. exp. Biol. Med.*, **68**, 1.

RUDDY, S., FEARON, D. T. and AUSTEN, K. F. (1975). *Arthr. and Rheum.*, **18**, 289.

SCHUMACHER, H. R. and KITRIDOU, R. C. (1972). *Arthr. and Rheum.*, **15**, 465.

SCHUR, P. and AUSTEN, F. (1971). *Bull. rheum. Dis.*, **22**, 666.

SHELDON, P. J., PAPAMICHAIL, M. and HOLBOROW, J. (1974). *Ann. rheum. Dis.*, **33**, 509.

SINGER, J. M. (1961). *Amer. J. Med.*, **31**, 766.

SMILEY, J. D., SACKS, C. and ZIFF, M. (1968). *J. clin. Invest.*, **47**, 624.

STASTNY, P., ROSENTHAL, M., ANDREIS, M. and ZIFF, M. (1975). *Arthr. and Rheum.*, **18**, 237.

STEWART, S. M., ALEXANDER, W. R. M. and DUTHIE, J. J. R. (1969). *Ann. Rheum. Dis.*, **28**, 477.

TANNENBAUM, H. and SCHUR, P. H. (1974). *J. Rheumatol.*, **1**, 392.

TANNENBAUM, H., PINCUS, G. S., ANDERSON, L. G. and SCHUR, P. (1975). *Arthr. and Rheum.*, **18**, 30.

VAN BOXEL, J. A. and PAGET, S. A. (1975). *New Engl. J. Med.*, **293**, 517.

VERSEY, J. M. B., HOBBS, J. R. and HOLT, P. J. L. (1973). *Ann. Rheum. Dis.*, **32**, 557.

WEINSTEIN, A., PETERS, K., BROWN, D. and BLUESTONE, R. (1972). *Arthr. and Rheum.*, **15**, 49.

WEISMAN, M. and ZVAIFLER, N. (1975). *J. clin. Invest.*, **56**, 725.

WHALEY, K., GLEN, A. C. A., MACSWEEN, R. N. M., DEODHAR, S., DICK, W. C., NUKI, G., WILLIAMSON, J. and BUCHANAN, W. W. (1971). *Clin. exp. Immunol.*, **9**, 721.

WILLIAMS, M. H., BROSTOFF, J. and ROITT, I. M. (1970). *Lancet*, **2**, 277.

WILLIAMS, R. C., EMMONS, J. D. and YUNIS, E. J. (1971). *J. clin. Invest.*, **50**, 1514.

WILLIAMS, R. C., DEBOARD, J. R., MELLBYE, O. J., MESSNER, R. P., LINDSTROM, F. D. (1973). *J. clin. Invest.*, **52**, 283.

WINCHESTER, R. J., KUNKEL, H. G. and AGNELLO, V. (1971). *J. exp. Med.*, **134**, 286 (s).

WINCHESTER, R. J., SIEGAL, F. P., BENTWICH, Z. H. and KUNKEL, H. G. (1973). *Arthr. and Rheum.*, **16**, 138.

WINCHESTER, R. J., FU, S. M., HOFFMAN, T., WINFIELD, J. B. and KUNKEL, H. G. (1975). In *Immunological Basis of Connective Tissue Disorders*. Ed. L. G. Silvestri. North Holland Publishing Co., Amsterdam.

YATES, D. B. and SCOTT, J. T. (1975). *Ann. rheum. Dis.*, **34**, 1.

ZVAIFLER, N. (1973). *Adv. Immunol.*, **16**, 265.

6

Systemic Lupus Erythematosus

Introduction

Systemic lupus erythematosus (SLE) is a multi-system disorder most commonly affecting young women, characterized by the presence of autoantibodies directed against cellular nuclear constituents. Polyarthritis or polyarthralgia occur in almost all patients with SLE, together with simultaneous or episodic and phasic involvement of skin, kidneys, haemopoietic tissue, lung, heart, blood vessels and the nervous system, as well as non-specific symptoms such as fever, malaise and weight loss. Spontaneous remissions and exacerbations are usual, a relatively benign course being more frequent than was formerly appreciated (for a review of natural history see Estes and Christian, 1971), but the disease may be fatal, with an estimated mortality rate of around 50 per cent at 10 years; renal failure, neurological complications and infection are important causes of death (reviewed by Dubois, 1974).

Although the aetiology of SLE remains unknown, the emergence of obvious autoimmune phenomena so characteristic of the disease, indicates a failure of the regulatory mechanisms which in health prevent an immune response from occurring against 'self' antigens. Apart from their undoubted value in the diagnosis and management of patients with SLE, the presence of autoantibodies appears to be of major pathogenetic significance, for example, in the production of auto-allergic damage to cells, and in immune complex-mediated connective tissue and vascular lesions. In this chapter, the basis for the belief that multi-system involvement has an immune pathogenesis will be examined by reviewing the information that has accumulated from studies of tissues and body fluids. The detection of autoantibodies in this disease and their clinical significance will also be discussed.

Joint disease

The joints are frequently involved with SLE, the typical lesion being a non-erosive synovitis with little deformity. When deformities do occur they tend to be of the rare type described by Jaccoud following rheumatic fever, in which ulnar deviation and subluxation of the metacarpophalangeal (MCP) joints or hyper-extension of the proximal interphalangeal (PIP) joints can sometimes be corrected by appropriate passive or voluntary movement. The synovial changes have not been extensively studied, but proliferation of the synovial lining layer and infiltration of the subsynovium with mononuclear cells are not as marked as that usually seen in rheumatoid arthritis (Labowitz and Schumacher, 1971). Ultrastructural studies have shown intracytoplasmic tubular inclusions in the endothelial cells of synovial blood vessels. A fibrotic subsynovium with sparse mononuclear infiltration has been described. Our own experience suggests that in acute phases of arthritis in SLE, usually lasting a few days, there is an exudative synovitis with dilated blood vessels and perivascular mononuclear cell infiltration but plasma cells do not appear.

The synovial fluid in SLE is usually clear and contains a sparse number of mononuclear cells, rarely exceeding 2,000 per cubic millimetre. The protein content in one study was found to be sometimes low, suggesting that the effusion was a transudate, possibly due to increased capillary permeability, whereas in other patients the protein level was raised in keeping with an exudate, presumably arising as a result of an inflammatory response (Pekin and Zvaifler, 1970). Complement levels in the joint fluid were reported to be low in those synovial fluids with protein contents suggestive of transudates, but since the serum complement levels of these patients were also low, it was thought likely that the low synovial fluid levels reflected changes in blood. In other patients (in this and another study, Hedberg, 1967), clinically characterized as having chronic arthritis in conjunction with SLE, the synovial fluid was an exudate (with a raised protein content), and showed lower complement levels than in the blood, suggesting local utilization in the joint. Only very low levels of IgM or IgG rheumatoid factor were detected in the synovial fluid of some patients in these studies; and it seems unlikely that IgG rheumatoid factor complexes, of the type present in abundance in rheumatoid effusions, are responsible for low complement levels found in SLE.

Kidney

The kidney in SLE may be involved in up to 60 per cent of patients, depending on the criteria and selection of patients (reviewed by Pollack and Pirani, 1974). Using light microscopy the changes have been classified basically into four types: (1) minimal change with some hypertrophy of the mesangium; (2) membranous glomerulonephritis; (3) focal glomerulonephritis in which changes are confined to some glomeruli, the rest being normal; (4) diffuse glomerulonephritis with all glomeruli involved. Other criteria are used for defining active, as opposed to inactive, disease. These changes have been reviewed by Pollak and Pirani, and carry a certain prognostic significance, the first two types being associated with a relatively good prognosis (20 per cent mortality at 5 years), the third with an intermediate prognosis and the fourth type with the worst outlook, the majority of patients (treated with low doses of steroids) dying from renal failure or its complications within 2 years. In general, the character and severity of the renal disease are established early and remain 'true to type' (Zveiman *et al.*, 1968) although changes from one pattern to another may occur rarely in the same patient. On the other hand, patients whose kidneys remain free of involvement during the early stages of the disease rarely develop significant renal disease at a later stage.

The concept that the renal abnormalities in lupus are a consequence of immune complex deposition has arisen largely from immunofluorescent and ultrastructural studies on biopsy materials as well as from examination of kidneys obtained at autopsy. Using immunofluorescent techniques, renal biopsies with little or no change on light microscopy may show IgG deposits in the mesangium, and occasionally C3 as well (Morel-Maroger *et al.*, 1971). Electron microscopy of such biopsies is said to frequently show minor changes in the basement membrane of glomeruli. In the membranous type of SLE nephritis, the entire glomerular basement membrane (GBM) appears thickened with deposits staining for immunoglobulin and complement. The deposits lie within the substance of the GBM or on its outer aspect beneath the epithelial cells (a situation termed subepithelial or epimembranous), with 'spikes' of basement membrane interdigitating with the deposits. Linear staining of the GBM appearing as a homogeneous band, resembling the appearance of the glomerulus in Goodpasture's syndrome, is rarely seen, and is distinguishable from it by the absence of complement staining in SLE. This pattern is usually seen in the presence of little or no renal functional abnormality (Agnello *et al.*, 1973), in complete contrast to the usually severe impairment of renal function in Goodpasture's syndrome. Granular and 'lumpy-bumpy' deposits on the GBM are observed by immunofluorescent techniques when glomerulonephritis is active or when renal disease is advanced (see Fig. 6.1). Electron microscopy of these sections shows that granular and lumpy deposits may be subendothelial in their distribution or may lie within the GBM giving rise to an appearance of 'splitting'; in most instances electron-dense material is also found in other areas of the kidney. Electron microscopy may also show the presence of endothelial cytoplasmic microtubular structures resembling paramyxoviruses (Gyorkey *et al.*, 1969) as well as other details such as the fusion of foot processes, electron-dense deposits in the mesangium and increase of the mesangial matrix.

The finding of complement together with immunoglobulin in deposits on the GBM has been taken to indicate that complement is involved in the production of the renal lesion. By using specific antisera it has been demonstrated that C3 is deposited in the GBM in the majority of cases of renal SLE, and C1q is found in 60–80 per cent of the biopsies (Lewis *et al.*, 1970; Koffler *et al.*, 1974). These findings have raised the possibility that complement activation may occur via the classical pathway in the majority of patients; it is probably mediated by DNA–anti-DNA antibody complexes as well as other polynucleotide–antibody systems which have been demonstrated in the kidney. The finding of properdin (Michael and McLean, 1974) in some of the biopsies has also implicated the alternate pathway although it is not clear whether this mechanism is preferentially involved in some patients or whether it merely serves to amplify immune complex activation. Studies on blood complement levels suggest that both classical (Gewurtz *et al.*, 1968) and alternate pathways (Perrin *et al.*, 1975) are involved. The known ability of C1q to precipitate with DNA and the invariable association

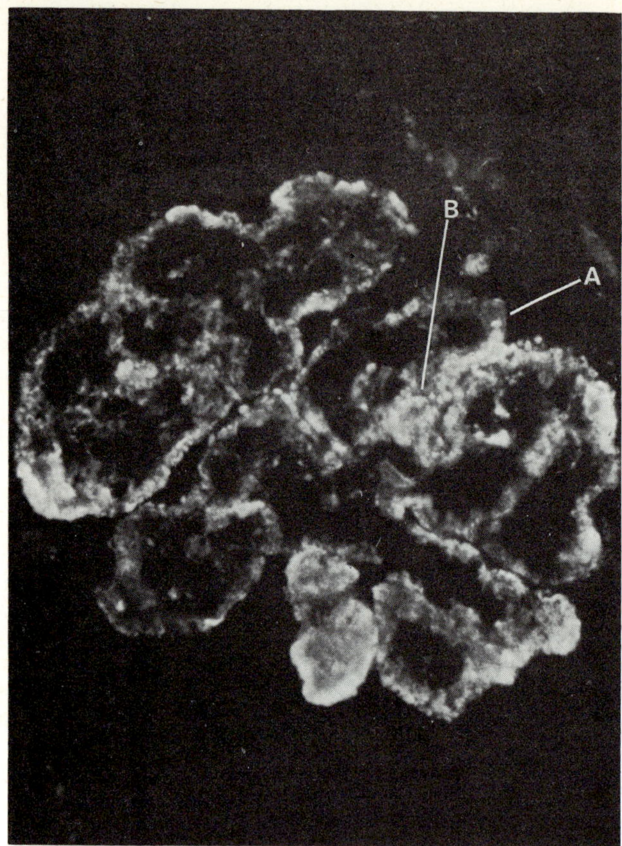

Fig. 6.1 Immunofluorescent staining with fluorescein-labelled anti-human IgG of a glomerulus from a patient with diffuse proliferative lupus nephritis. The gammaglobulin is distributed along the capillary loops (**A**) and in the mesangium (**B**) in a granular or globular pattern (magnification × 160; enlarged × 3.2).

of C1q with SS-DNA in kidneys (Koffler *et al.*, 1974) could indicate that complement activation might occur following binding to the antigen itself. The finding of IgM rheumatoid factor by immunofluorescence in tissue sections of kidneys from patients with severe SLE nephritis, and identification of rheumatoid factor of the same idiotypic specificity in the cryoglobulin-containing IgG-rheumatoid factor complexes, implicate an additional immune complex system in the nephritis of SLE (Agnello *et al.*, 1973).

The participation of immune complexes in renal SLE is further substantiated by elution studies of Koffler *et al.* (1974) in which a variety of polynucleotide antibodies, including antibodies to DS-DNA, SS-DNA and ribonuclear proteins, as well as the antigen SS-DNA, have been demonstrated.

Although hypocomplementaemia is also usually associated with disease activity (Schur and Sandson, 1968), it is not clear whether participation of complement is essential for the development of the immune complex renal lesions. In a study on SLE patients in which subclasses of IgG deposited in the kidney were determined, it was found that the predominant subclass was IgG2, which does not fix complement as avidly as IgG1 and IgG3 (Lewis *et al.*, 1970). In the experimental model of immune complex nephritis, renal lesions occur in spite of the total depletion of complement in the animals, indicating that, in this situation at least, complement is not essential.

The localization of complexes in the kidney in SLE resembles that seen in experimental chronic nephritis in rabbits induced by Dixon and his associates with heterologous serum proteins. In the experimental model, circulating complexes deposit on the GBM, and the factors which determine their localization include haemodynamic filtration pressure, the release of vasoactive amines by reaginic (IgE-sensitized) basophils by antigen, the size of the immune complexes, their ability to bind complement and the quality of the antibody response (Chapter 2). Another factor which might be expected to influence immune complex clearance is the phagocytic function of the reticuloendothelial system. The possibility that the glomerular mesangium contains cells that have phagocytic activity has been put forward; in experimental chronic nephritis some evidence of fatigue of these cells has been postulated (Wilson and Dixon, 1971), thus allowing accumulation and deposition of immune complexes on the GBM following saturation of the mesangium and their overflow between the endothelial cells and the GBM. The importance of these factors in animal models and SLE requires clarification.

Central nervous system

The pathological basis of the neurological disorder requires further documentation, but consists at least to some extent of vascular disease with occlusions of small arteries causing infarcts, or haemorrhages (reviewed by Johnson and Richardson, 1968). The increased occurrence of anti-neuronal (cytoplasmic) antibodies (Quismorio and Friou, 1972) in patients with central nervous system (CNS) involvement seemed much more frequent than in patients in whom the CNS was not involved, but since the reaction was also observed with a cytoplasmic constituent of other organs, the antibody belongs to the 'non-organ-specific' class and is unlikely to be an important factor in localization to the CNS. However, it was found that 41 per cent of patients with SLE and CNS manifestations had such antibodies, compared with 9 per cent of SLE patients without CNS disease. In another report of 2 patients with SLE, who died as a result of neurological complications, examination of the choroid plexus of the brain by immunofluorescent techniques showed deposition of IgM in both, and IgG in one. Electron-dense deposits were found between the vascular and epithelial parts of the basement membrane, and resembled deposits seen in the kidney (Atkins *et al.*, 1972). The possibility that a rise of IgM–anti-DNA antibody in amounts equivalent to IgG antibody may be implicated in CNS disease has been suggested by preliminary findings in patients with obvious organic neurological manifestations in SLE (Griffiths *et al.*, 1976). The occurrence of precipitating antibodies detected by a counter-immunoelectrophoresis test was more frequent in patients with CNS disease and vasculitis than in those without (Johnson *et al.*, 1973).

Abnormally low levels of C4 components of complement in the cerebrospinal fluid of patients with SLE was found in one study (Petz *et al.*, 1971), although a later investigation showed that random determinations of C4 levels in the CSF were not of diagnostic value, since the component was unstable, and levels varied greatly from patient to patient and overlapped with the values found in patients who did not have CNS involvement (Hadler *et al.*, 1973). However, in individual patients sequential studies did show a significant drop in the level of C4, suggesting that complement activation by immune complexes may be involved in the pathogenesis of cerebral manifestations.

Circulating antibodies may therefore be of pathogenetic significance in CNS manifestations, and complement activation may occur in this process during the acute stages of the disease.

Skin manifestations

The skin is often involved, erythema characteristically affecting the 'butterfly area' of the face, also the extremities and trunk. Other types of lesions include urticaria, bullae and maculopapular lesions, ulceration and alopecia of the scalp (which is common during active phases of the disease). Exposure to sunlight can cause erythema or more severe burns, and experimental exposure of skin to monochromatic light has induced 'lupus' lesions. Examination of involved skin by light microscopy shows degeneration of the deep epidermal layers as well as necrotic changes in the dermal fibroblasts and a variable degree of vascular change, including perivascular mononuclear cell infiltration and fibrinoid change in the vessel wall.

Studies using immunofluorescent techniques have drawn attention to the presence of immunoglobulin and complement deposition in the dermoepidermal junction and in the vessel walls (Tan and Kunkel, 1966). The deposit in the dermoepidermal junction has been reported to occur in clinically involved skin in patients with SLE and chronic discoid lupus, but other disorders, including dermatomyositis and other skin disorders, may show similar changes so that the appearance is not specific. However, the finding of immunoglobulin and complement deposits in clinically uninvolved skin has been found in up to 50 per cent of patients with SLE and appears to correlate with the immunofluorescent changes found in the kidney, and to this extent may provide an accessible means of monitoring renal disease activity (Gilliam *et al.*, 1974). The origin of the immune deposits is not clear, but it has been suggested that they could represent interaction of nuclear antigens released from necrotic epidermal cells reacting with anti-nuclear antibodies present in the circulation, rather than a result of deposition of pre-formed circulating complexes. Anti-nuclear antibodies as well as anti-basement-membrane antibodies have been eluted from skin (Landry and Sams, 1973), the significance of the latter being ill understood. Some biopses of, skin from SLE patients show IgG bound to the nuclei of epidermal cells, suggesting an *in vivo* reaction of unknown significance.

Vascular disease

Fibrinoid degeneration and arteritis are observed in various organs and systems; for example, renal arteries and arterioles. In addition, digital vessels are frequently involved, as indicated by Raynaud's phenomenon, or by more serious ischaemic changes, necrosis and gangrene. Attention has been drawn to the prevalence of precipitating, non-complement-fixing DNA antibodies with vasculitis, as well as to very high levels of anti-nuclear antibodies. The demonstration of immuno-globulin and complement in the vessel walls has suggested the involvement of complexes in arteritic lesions, but it is not clear whether they account for all the pathological lesions seen in blood vessels, including the endarteritis seen in digital vessels.

Liver

Overt involvement of the liver is not common in typical cases of SLE with renal, neurological and other features. However, in active chronic hepatitis (lupoid hepatitis), presenting with jaundice and biochemical evidence of liver cell necrosis, anti-nuclear antibodies are often present in the blood. Anti-DNA antibodies have been found in active chronic hepatitis, which sometimes shows features of a multi-system disorder including the development of polyarteritis, renal tubular acidosis, Sjögren's syndrome and even changes on renal biopsy not dissimilar to lupus nephritis. The presence of smooth muscle antibody in this group of patients in the majority of cases contrasts with an incidence of 30 per cent in SLE, but does not differentiate an individual patient. Thus there are overlapping clinical, pathological and serological features between chronic active hepatitis, SLE and other autoimmune diseases.

Lungs

Pleurisy, pleural effusions, interstitial pneumonitis, and diffuse fibrosing alveolitis occur in SLE (Estes and Christian, 1971). Complement levels in pleural effusions in SLE (and rheumatoid arthritis) are reported to be reduced (Hunder *et al.*, 1972). The possibility that anti-nuclear antibodies may play a pathogenetic role has been investigated and it was shown that a chemical pleurisy in rats induced by intrapleural instillation of turpentine was accentuated by the simultaneous injection of anti-nuclear antibody (reviewed by Turner-Warwick, 1974). The finding of immune complexes within the mesothelial cells by these workers suggested that phagocytosis of immune complexes leading to release of lysosomal enzymes may be an important mechanism in the evolution of pleural pathology. This experiment suggested that in SLE, nuclear antigens from mesothelial debris may complex with circulating antibody, and the finding of intracellular inclusions in mesothelial cells in a single case of lupus with pleural effusion has been reported by Turner-Warwick.

Attention has been drawn to the serological features of idiopathic fibrosing alveolitis in which anti-nuclear antibodies and rheumatoid factors frequently occur, and conversely, to the well documented occurrence of a lung disorder in SLE, histopathologically indistinguishable from fibrosing alveolitis. The relationship between these diseases and their serological features remains uncertain, but immunofluorescent studies on a lung biopsy specimen showed evidence of complement and IgG in the alveolar capillaries of a patient with SLE. The possibility that the quality of antigen specificity of anti-nuclear antibodies may be important in the evolution of lung disorders was suggested by the results of a study of 22 patients with SLE presenting with lung symptoms, in whom DNA antibody detected by a precipitating technique was present in nearly all of them, but was detectable in only 25 per cent of them by the Farr assay (Holgate *et al.*, 1976).

Haematological abnormalities

Cell-bound or circulating antibody to red blood cells in SLE provides an example of a truly autoallergic antibody, since it mediates haemolysis of the red cells *in vivo*. The antibody may be detected by Coombs' antiglobulin agglutination tests, of either the direct or the indirect variety. In the former, anti-human globulin agglutinates red cells, although a specific autoantibody is not always demonstrable, and positive tests have been reported when red cells could only be shown to have bound complement (Mongan *et al.*, 1967). The indirect test detects serum antibody, and when associated with haemolytic anaemia tends to be of the 'warm' antibody type. The direct Coombs' test has been reported to be positive in 25–75 per cent in different series; however, it is associated with a haemolytic process in a smaller proportion of cases, sometimes, however, being a presenting feature (Estes and Christian, 1971).

Leucopenia is not uncommon in SLE, although its mechanism is unexplained. Leucocyte agglutinins or lymphocyte cytotoxins may be responsible. Blood granulocytes from SLE patients also show a decreased phagocytic function, and this defect appears to be independent of steroid therapy, but whether it involves serum factors is not certain.

Platelet antibodies have been detected in SLE in a large number of patients, although the tests used do not yet appear to be entirely reliable. There is little doubt that a 7S immunoglobulin is responsible for the thrombocytopenia sometimes found in SLE patients since infusion of SLE serum in normal individuals led to a depletion of platelet count of the recipient (Shulman *et al.*, 1965). The relationship of SLE to idiopathic thrombocytopenic purpura is interesting, since some of the patients with this disorder eventually develop features of SLE (Baldini, 1972).

Autoimmune serological phenomena

The occurrence of a number of antibodies directed against nuclear and cytoplasmic constituents in SLE is well documented (see Chapter 3). SLE is characteristically associated with the presence of a large number of LE cells and a high titre of anti-nuclear antibodies (a peripheral rim-type pattern on nuclear immunofluorescence being particularly specific, but much less common than the less specific homogeneous staining pattern). Measurements of antibodies to DS-DNA, especially by the Farr assay, have shown that raised levels tend to be confined to patients with SLE but are not exclusive to this condition (see Holian *et al.*, 1975, for references). The appearance of DNA antibody may precede clinical exacerbations, and the presence of DNA antibodies accompanied by lowered serum complement levels almost invariably indicates disease activity and is frequently associated with renal involvement (Schur and Sandson, 1968). However, patients with SLE can have active disease without evidence of circulating DS-DNA antibodies. In such patients sequential studies may show raised antibody levels alternating with circulating DNA antigen, suggesting that the antibodies may be bound in an immune complex which is either being rapidly cleared from blood by the reticuloendothelial system or being deposited in target organs such as the kidney (Koffler *et al.*, 1974). Antibodies to single-stranded DNA, although diagnostically much less specific for SLE, are nevertheless often present in active SLE, and have been extracted from affected kidneys even when circulating antibodies to SS-DNA could not be demonstrated. Antibodies to a soluble nuclear RNA-protein extract, also referred to as extractable nuclear antigens (ENA), were reported by one group of workers to be indicative of a less severe steroid-responsive form of renal lupus, as well as being characteristic of a syndrome termed 'mixed connective tissue disease' (Chapter 3). However, in Koffler's study this antibody was found in high concentrations in the blood, often alternating with antigen, but only the antibody could be eluted from the kidney, suggesting that this system of immune complex may not be implicated in damage of the kidney.

Among the various antibody derangements in SLE, one of particular clinical interest is the so-called 'chronic biologic false-positive' test for syphilis in which a positive serological test for syphilis may be found in SLE, sometimes preceding clinical signs of the disease by many years. Anti-nuclear factors have been found in up to 50 per cent of such sera (Johansson *et al.*, 1972).

Immune complexes and complement

Several lines of evidence suggest that immune complexes circulate in the serum prior to their deposition on the glomerular basement membrane in SLE. Lowering of serum complement levels corresponds with periods of disease activity. The following observations indicate the importance of immune complexes in SLE.

1. The demonstration of nuclear antigen alternating with antibody; e.g. antibodies to DS-DNA, SS-DNA and RNA-protein alternating with the demonstration of the corresponding polynucleotide antigen (Koffler *et al.*, 1974). These findings suggest that immune complexes formed in antigen equivalence or excess are involved in the renal disease, as documented in experimental chronic nephritis in rabbits.

2. The direct demonstration of polynucleotides and their antibodies in kidneys by immunofluorescent and elution studies on the kidneys (see section on 'Kidney', earlier in this chapter).

3. Depletion of total haemolytic complement and early components C1, 4, 2 and 3 is not uncommon in SLE and suggests activation by immune complexes. However, activation of the alternate pathway which has also been shown to occur, must contribute to the reduction of the total haemolytic complement activity and C3, and the mechanism of its activation in this disease is not clear. Moreover, evidence has been put forward that synthesis of certain complement components may be congenitally depleted in some patients with SLE (Chapter 13). Thus the finding of lowered complement levels is not always an indication of immune complex formation *in vivo*, and should be interpreted with caution.

4. The presence of cryoprecipitates, composed of the C1q component of complement, IgM and IgG (the immunoglobulin showing rheumatoid factor activity) in active disease suggest participation of immune complexes of IgG–anti-IgG in the pathogenesis of SLE. The demonstration by Agnello *et al.*, (1973) that IgG rheumatoid factor deposits were present in the kidneys in SLE patients with cryoprecipitates in the serum further suggests that these immune complexes are implicated in renal damage. However, low levels of rheumatoid factors in SLE are not uncommon and do not appear to be always associated with more severe disease or renal involvement. Although the presence of cryoprecipitates usually runs parallel with raised serum anti-DNA antibodies, this is not necessarily the case. A recent study has, however, shown enrichment of anti-polynucleotide antibodies in cryoprecipitates (Winfield *et al.*, 1975).

5. The precipitation of immune complexes and aggregated IgG with C1q in gel has been used as a test for complexes in SLE. Two-thirds of hypocomplementaemic sera gave positive reactions in a study by Agnello *et al.* (1971). The C1q reactants appeared to be either of high molecular weight ($>19S$), in which case their composition resembled that of cryoprecipitates obtained from the same sera (see above), or were of a molecular size in the region of 7–10S. The low molecular weight complexes consist of immunoglobulin bound to unidentified molecules, possibly including materials of exogenous origin and of aetiological importance. A recently developed technique using radio-labelled C1q precipitation with polyethylene glycol (Nyedegger *et al.*, 1974) has confirmed the findings of C1q reactants in the sera of patients with SLE. This test, however, is positive not only in SLE but also in patients with rheumatoid arthritis and Australia antigen hepatitis in distinction to the precipitation in agar, possibly indicating its greater sensitivity.

6. In a study on sera of patients with SLE with anti-DNA antibodies, it was shown that the amount of anti-DNA antibody activity increased after treatment of the serum with DNAse, thus indicating release of some antibody which was presumed to be previously bound to DNA (Harbeck *et al.*, 1973). Apart from this single study, however, no direct evidence has been forthcoming which has identified anti-DNA antibody complexed to DNA in the serum of these patients. The likely explanation of this finding is that such complexes, formed in antibody excess, are of a type which are usually rapidly cleared by the reticuloendothelial system.

7. IgG-rich pellets which reacted with C1q in agar were separated by high-speed centrifugation of SLE sera in sucrose gradients (Bombardieri *et al.*, 1973). The pellets could not be dissociated at low pH, and therefore are unlike immune complexes.

Lymphocyte subpopulations

Circulating blood lymphocytes have been noted to be reduced in absolute numbers in many patients with SLE, especially when the disease is active. Although in an initial study the percentage of T cells in SLE patients was reported to be similar to those of controls, a later study from the same group reported that the T cell population, enumerated by two separate techniques utilizing anti-T cell antisera and E-rosettes, was reduced both in absolute numbers and as a percentage of the total lymphocyte population in patients with active disease (Messner *et al.*, 1973). A wide fluctuation in T cell numbers was also noted in serial studies and far exceeded that observed in controls. Reduction in T cells has also been reported by other workers. The possibility has been suggested that T cell depletion is related to the presence of lymphocytotoxic antibodies in blood. However, these antibodies occur much more commonly than actual lymphopenia in SLE; they have also been noted in a large proportion of relatives and unrelated family members living with SLE patients (De Horatius and Messner, 1975).

Enumeration of B cells in blood has produced inconsistent results. Using the technique of immunofluorescent staining for surface Ig, a significant increase in the percentage of such cells compared with healthy control subjects was noted by Messner *et al.* (1973), although the absolute number was still significantly lower than that of healthy controls. The total and percentage of cells were diminished when B cells were detected by EAC-rosette tests. In another study using erythrocytes coated with F (ab^1)$_2$ for a rosette test for B cells, no difference between SLE and controls was observed. The possible reasons for the discrepancies is discussed in the chapter on Immunological Methods (Chapter 4); for example, in a more recent study on SLE patients which took into account some of the more important variables, T cells were found to be slightly increased and Ig-positive cells diminished compared to controls (Winchester *et al.*, 1974). The studies must be regarded as inconclusive so far.

Immune status

Impairment of delayed hypersensitivity reactions to ubiquitous antigens has been reported to be depressed in most studies, although there is a lack of agreement on details. Depressed reactions to tuberculin PPD has been generally observed; reactions to Candida, trichophytin, SKSD and histoplasmin were similarly depressed except in one study in which they were found to be comparable to normals (reviewed by Tennebaum and Schur, 1974). It should be noted that in this study no differences between SLE and controls were found to PPD, trichophytin and histoplasmin. The ability to acquire contact sensitization to dinitrochlorobenzene has been reported to be depressed in SLE patients, indicating a defect of cellular immunity (Abe and Homma, 1971). As in rheumatoid arthritis, it appears that total anergy to antigens is unusual and the extent of depression of delayed hypersensitivity is not uniform. No reliable information exists concerning the relationship in the tests to the age of the patient, the past immune status, the duration of disease, its activity, whether the disease involves one or more systems or whether drug treatment has been taken into account. Even allowing for such factors the quantitative aspects of the acquisition and maintenance of delayed hypersensitivity to antigens is presumably a very individual experience, and is difficult to compare with controls. It was for this reason that the report of a depressed delayed hypersensitivity reaction to antigens as well as a diminished acquisition of delayed hypersensitivity to KLH in a patient with SLE compared with her identical healthy twin seemed especially significant (Horwitz, 1972). However, these studies leave unanswered the question of whether the depressed reactions result from the disease itself or were present as an important pre-existing defect of cellular immunity.

Lymphocyte transformation tests with PHA (see review by Tannenbaum and Schur, 1974) have been predictably reported to cover all possibilities. Thus, compared with controls, there was no difference to PHA, increased responses to PHA and depressed responses to PHA. The possibility exists that in those studies in which *in vitro* tests were performed in the presence of autologous serum, or in those studies in which steps were not taken to carefully wash the cells free of serum, the results may have shown a depression of lymphocyte response because of the frequent occurrence of lymphocytotoxic antibody; in addition, a non-cytotoxic IgG fraction of SLE serum which depresses PHA responses has been reported. It is likely, however, that lack of agreement in the results is mainly ascribable to lack of standardization of the tests with the additional possibility that PHA responsiveness of lymphocytes in patients with SLE may be more variable and cover a wider range of responses than in healthy controls, analogous to the situation noted by us in a study in rheumatoid arthritis (Maini *et al.*, 1976). A widely fluctuating number of T cells in peripheral blood was noted in SLE patients in one study (Messner *et al.*, 1973), and suggests that results of lymphocyte transformation might be less variable if they were expressed in relation to absolute T cell counts.

Infective aetiological theory

There are compelling reasons for believing that viruses are of aetiological importance in SLE although so far the evidence in largely indirect (reviewed by Ziff, 1971). Much of it arises from comparison with experimental observations on mice and other animals, which indicate that a virus infection is responsible for the appearance of anti-nuclear antibodies (ANA) and an immune-complex glomerulonephritis which has remarkable similarities to SLE. Thus in New Zealand (NZ) mice of the 'black' variety and in the hybrid offspring of 'black and white' strains, Mellors and Huang (1966) found evidence of infection with a RNA virus of the type normally associated with an oncogenic potential in producing leukaemia or lymphoma. These so-called oncorna viruses (of type C) have been isolated from lymphoblastoid-cell lines from NZ mice. When injected in a viable form they accelerate naturally occurring disease in NZ mice; moreover, when injected into a variety of strains of mice, they lead to the appearance of anti-nuclear antibodies sometimes accompanied by an immune-complex nephritis, whereas these strains do not normally show such features (Dixon *et al.*, 1974). The amount of ANA frequently, but not always, parallels the severity of nephritis, depending on the genetic composition of the animals.

A type C virus has also been implicated in an SLE syndrome in a specially bred colony of dogs (Lewis *et al.*, 1973). The virus hypothesis has been further elaborated by this group of workers in Boston and it has been claimed that cell-free filtrates of lymphoid tissue from affected dogs induces a lupus syndrome in murine recipient strains, but attempts to demonstrate viral material in these filtrates have proven unsuccessful. It is therefore possible that cell-free filtrate induces activation of a dormant murine oncogenic virus. A specific antiserum prepared against the C-type virus in pigs was shown to react with the surface membranes of a proportion of circulating lymphocytes of human SLE patients, suggesting the presence of C-type antigens presumably as a result of infection with oncorna virus (Schwartz, 1975).

The finding by electron microscopy of interwoven tubular structures in the cytoplasm of renal glomerular endothelial cells was interpreted by Gyorkey *et al.*, (1969) as representing viral material resembling the nucleocapsids of paramyxoviruses of the type seen in brain tissue of patients with subacute sclerosing panencephalitis, thought to be a measles virus infection (reviewed by Christian and Phillips, 1973). Similar tubular structures have also been found in circulating lymphocytes of patients with SLE (Klippel *et al.*, 1974), as well as in the skin of patients with discoid lupus. The finding is not specific for lupus as the same structure has been found in a variety of tissues from patients with Sjögren's syndrome, polymyositis, lymphomas, Goodpasture's syndrome and rheumatoid arthritis. Serious doubts have been expressed as to the viral nature of these structures, attention being drawn to similar appearances in lymphoid cells of patients with the genetically inherited disease of metabolism, cystinosis (Pincus *et al.*, 1970). The tubular structures do not resemble the type-C inclusions observed in the experimental models of SLE, although host response could alter the morphological appearance of the virus.

Other evidence sometimes cited in favour of a viral aetiology is the finding of raised serum antibody levels to viruses in SLE. However, antibodies are raised to both RNA- and DNA-type viruses (e.g. measles, rubella, herpes simplex and Epstein–Barr virus), and a simple relationship to the serum globulin level, indicating a non-specific type of response, has been suggested (see Christian and Phillips, 1973). The finding of raised anti-viral antibodies in other diseases such as sarcoidosis, rheumatoid arthritis and multiple sclerosis casts further doubts on their specific significance. Antibodies to synthetic and viral double-stranded RNA in SLE were thought to indicate a more specific response to replicating virus, since only the single-stranded form of this nucleic acid occurs in mammalian tissues (Schur *et al.*, 1971) but the immunological specificity of the reaction requires confirmation and immunological hyper-reactivity to ubiquitous double-stranded RNA virus is an additional possibility. In contrast to elevated antibody titres to a variety of viruses, diminished cellular hypersensitivity specifically directed against measles antigen using a migration inhibition test has been described (Utermohlen *et al.*, 1974).

The finding of lymphocytotoxic antibodies in patients with SLE has suggested the possibility of a virus-induced loss of tolerance to autoantigens (Terasaki *et al.*, 1970; and see Chapter 1) and its finding in non-consanguinous members of the family of patients with SLE has suggested a possible infective 'horizontal' transmission of virus (DeHoratius and Messner, 1975).

In a recently published report, DNA extracted from a lymph node, kidney and leucocytes of a patient with SLE was shown to contain DNA sequences homologous with the RNA of measles virus, and cytoplasmic extracts contained reverse transcriptase activity of the type seen in cells infected with oncorna viruses (Zhdanov, 1975). On the basis of this observation it was suggested that in certain rare cases of infection with measles, a latent oncorna virus might provide the reverse transcriptase activity required for the transcription of measles virus RNA into double-stranded DNA of the cell genome. Subsequently, the integrated viral genome may express virus-specific antigens on the host cell membrane and initiate autoimmunity. This study emphasizes the newly emerging concept of co-operation between infectious and oncogenic viruses and interactions with cells and the immune system in the pathogenesis of SLE.

Relationship between chronic discoid and systemic lupus erythematosus

Chronic discoid lupus erythematosus (CDLE) is primarily a skin disease and is characterized by the presence of plaques showing varying degrees of oedema, erythema, papular or depressed scaly lesions, follicular plugging, skin atrophy and telangiectasia surrounded by an elevated erythematous border. The face and scalp are usually affected, but occasionally widely disseminated (cutaneous) lesions occur. The 'butterfly area' (bridge of nose and cheeks) of the face, may be affected, and the clinical and histological appearance of the skin involvement are indistinguishable from those observed in a proportion (30 per cent) of patients with SLE. In general, however, patients with SLE predominantly show erythema with or without a maculopapular element, with minimal follicular plugging, scaling and skin atrophy.

Patients with CDLE do not as a rule develop serious systemic manifestations. Genetic differences between patients with CDLE and those with SLE have been suspected and this may explain the different features in the two groups of patients (Swanson Beck and Rowell, 1966). However, there are a number of arguments for regarding the two conditions either as closely related or as one and the same disease with CDLE as a localized (and often solitary) clinically overt manifestation of the same disorder. In several published series (reviewed by Dubois, 1974) patients with CDLE, sometimes of many years' duration, have been noted to develop multi-system manifestations of SLE. Furthermore, 13–26 per cent of patients with SLE, in two separate series, suffered from typical CDLE lesions at some stage of their disease (Tuffanelli and Dubois, 1964; Estes and Christian, 1971). The dividing line between CDLE on the one hand, and SLE on the other, may in any event be arbitrary since closer scrutiny of localized forms may show evidence of systemic manifestations which have escaped initial clinical detection (Dubois, 1974).

Serum from patients with CDLE not infrequently shows a positive test for anti-nuclear antibodies (35 per cent of cases described by Swanson Beck and Rowell, 1966) although the LE cell test is only rarely positive. Antibodies to double-stranded DNA were noted in a study in low amounts (Mandel *et al.*, 1972) and may be regarded as being somewhat more specific for SLE than immunofluorescent tests for anti-nuclear antibodies. Immunofluorescent studies on skin biopsies from patients with CDLE show a band of Ig and C3 deposition at the dermoepidermal junction identical to that observed in SLE. If clinically normal skin is biopsied, a large proportion of patients with active SLE show similar deposits (see earlier section on skin in SLE) whereas skin of CDLE patients does not (Tuffanelli *et al.*, 1969). These observations emphasize the similarities and differences between the two conditions which may be related to the presence of circulating complexes in SLE perhaps not usually present in CDLE.

The finding of tubuloreticular structures, possibly of viral origin, in skin biopsies of patients with CDLE resembles their occurrence in kidney biopsies of SLE patients (Grimley *et al.*, 1973). This finding could be regarded as providing evidence of a common aetiological agent, as can the finding of antibodies to viral and synthetic double-stranded RNA in 42 per cent of patients with CDLE (Sylvester *et al.*, 1973).

Drug-induced lupus erythematosus

Patients receiving a variety of drugs including hydrallazine, procainamide, isoniazid, D-penicillamine, chlorpromazine, anticonvulsants, methyldopa and practolol may develop anti-nuclear antibodies and anti-SS-DNA antibodies. A multi-system lupus syndrome is occasionally seen, especially following hydrallazine and procainamide (Alarcon-Segovia, 1969; Blomgren *et al.*, 1972), but renal involvement and hypocomplementaemia do not occur and antibodies to DS-DNA (which are usually present in active SLE) are not found in this syndrome. Patients on D-penicillamine therapy for rheumatoid arthritis and Wilson's disease also develop a similar syndrome (sometimes with renal involvement). In our laboratory, antibodies to DS-DNA have been recorded in 2 such non-renal cases (unpublished observations). Glomerulonephritis may also develop in some patients receiving D-penicillamine but is not usually part of a lupus syndrome and serum of such patients is usually negative for anti-nuclear antibodies.

As a rule, drug-induced lupus improves spontaneously following withdrawal of the drug. The mechanism of induction of autoimmunity is unknown and could include one of the several possibilities discussed in Chapter 1. Published theories emphasize the genetic aspects of a 'lupus diathesis', alteration by drugs of cellular constituents rendering them immunogenic, and activation of a latent virus. Some support for the hypothesis of alteration of nucleic acids by hydrallazine has been obtained in experimental studies (Blomgren *et al.*, 1972).

References

ABE, T. and HOMMA, M. (1971). *Acta rheum. scand.*, **17**, 35.

AGNELLO, V., KOFFLER, D., EISENBERG, J. W., WINCHESTER, R. J. and KUNKEL, H. G. (1971). *J. exp. Med.*, **134**, 228s.

AGNELLO, V., KOFFLER, D. and KUNKEL, H. G. (1973). *Kidney Int.*, **3**, 90.

ALARCON-SEGOVIA, D. (1969). *Mayo Clin. Proc.*, **44**, 664.

ATKINS, C. J., KONDON, J. J., QUISMORIO, F. P. and FRIOU, G. J. (1972). *Ann. Intern. Med.*, **76**, 65.

BALDINI, M. G. (1972). *Med. Clin. N. Amer.*, **56**, 47.

BLOMGREN, S. E., CONDEMI, J. J. and VAUGHAN, J. H. (1972). *Amer. J. Med.*, **52**, 338.

BOMBARDIERI, S., LIGHTFOOT, R. W., and CHRISTIAN, C. L. (1973). *Proc. Soc. exp. Biol. Med.*, **144**, 148.

CHRISTIAN, C. L. and PHILLIPS, P. E. (1973). *Amer. J. Med.*, **54**, 611.

DE HORATIUS, R. J. and MESSNER, R. P. (1975). *J. clin. Invest.*, **55**, 1254.

DIXON, F., CROKER, B., DELVILLANO, B., JENSEN, F. and LERNER, R. (1974). In *Progress in Immunology*, Vol. II, 5. Ed. L. Brent and J. Holborow. North Holland Publishing Co., Amsterdam.

DUBOIS, E. L. (1974). In *Lupus Erythematosus*, 2nd edn., pp. 455, 633. Ed. E. L. Dubois. University of Southern California Press, Berkeley.

ESTES, D. and CHRISTIAN, C. L. (1971). *Medicine (Baltimore)*, **50**, 85.

GEWURTZ, H., PICKERING, R. J., MERGENHAGEN, S. G. and GOOD, R. A. (1968). *Int. Arch. Allergy appl. Immunol.*, **34**, 556.

GILLIAM, J. N., CHEATUM, D. E., HURD, E. R., STASTNY, P. and ZIFF, M. (1974). *J. clin. Invest.*, **53**, 1434.

GRIFFITHS, I. D., GLASS, D. N., MANI, R. N. and SCOTT, J. T. (1976). *Ann. rheum. Dis.* (in press).

GRIMLEY, P. M., DECKER, J. L., MICHELITCH, H. J. and FRANTZ, M. M. (1973). *Arthr. and Rheum.*, **16**, 313.

GYORKEY, F., MIN, K. W., SINCOVIES, J. G. and GYORKEY, P. (1969). *New Engl. J. Med.*, **280**, 333.

HADLER, N. M., GERWIN, R. D., FRANK, M. M., WHITAKER, J. N., BAKER, M. and DECKER, J. L. (1973). *Arthr. and Rheum.*, **16**, 507.

HARBECK, R. J., BARDANA, E. J., KOHLER, P. F and CARR, R. I. (1973). *J. clin. Invest.*, **52**, 789.

HEDBERG, H. L. (1967). *Acta med. scand.* (Suppl.), **479**, 1.

HOLGATE, S. T., GLASS, D. N., HASLAM, P., MAINI, R. N. and TURNER-WARWICK, M. (1976). *Clin. exp. Immunol.*, **24**, 385.

HOLIAN, J., GRIFFITHS, I., GLASS, D. N., MAINI, R. N. and SCOTT, J. T. (1975). *Ann. rheum. Dis.*, **34**, 438.

HORWITZ, D. A. (1972). *Arthr. and Rheum.*, **15**, 353.

HUNDER, G. G., MCDUFFIE, F. C. and HEPPER, N. G. G. (1972). *Ann. intern. Med.*, **76**, 357.

JOHANSSON, E. A., LASSUS, A. and SALO, O. D. (1972). *Acta derm.-venereol. (Stockh.)*, **52**, 96.

JOHNSON, R. T. and RICHARDSON, E. P. (1968). *Medicine (Baltimore)*, **47**, 337.

JOHNSON, G. D., EDMONDS, J. P. and HOLBOROW, E. J. (1973). *Lancet*, **2**, 883.

KLIPPEL, J. H., GRIMLEY, P. M., DECKER, J. L. and MICHELITCH, H. J. (1974). *Ann. intern. Med.*, **81**, 355.

KOFFLER, D., AGNELLO, V. and KUNKEL, H. G. (1974). *Amer. J. Path.*, **74**, 109.

LABOWITZ, R. and SCHUMACHER, H. R. (1971). *Ann. intern. Med.*, **74**, 911.

LANDRY, M. and SAMS, Z. W. M. Jr. (1973). *J. clin. Invest.*, **52**, 1871.

LEWIS, E. J., BUSCH, G. J. and SCHUR, P. H. (1970). *J. clin. Invest.*, **49**, 1103.

LEWIS, R. M., ANDRE-SCHWARTZ, J., HARRIS, G. S., HIRSCH, M. S., BLACK, P. H. and SCHWARTZ, R. S. (1973). *J. clin. Invest.*, **52**, 1893.

MAINI, R. N., SCOTT, J. T., ROFFE, L., HAMBLIN, A. and DUMONDE, D. C. (1976). In *Infection and Immunity*, p. 579. Ed. D. C. Dumonde Blackwell Scientific, Oxford.

MANDEL, M. J., CARR, R. I., WESTON, W. L., SAMS, W. M., Jr. and HARBECK, R. J. (1972). *Arch. Derm.*, **106**, 668.

MELLORS, R. C. and HUANG, C. Y. (1966). *J. exp. Med.*, **124**, 1031.

MESSNER, R. P., LINDSTROM, F. D. and WILLIAMS, R. C. (1973). *J. clin. Invest.*, **52**, 3046.

MICHAEL, A. F. and MCLEAN, R. H. (1974). *Adv. Nephrol.*, **4**, 49.

MONGAN, E. S., LEDDY, J. P., ATWATER, E. C. and BARNETT, E. V. (1967). *Arthr. and Rheum.*, **10**, 502.

MOREL-MAROGER, L., MERY, J. PH., DELRIEU, F. and RICHET, G. (1971). *J. Urol. Néphrol. (Paris)*, **77**, 367.

NYEDEGGER, V. E., LAMBERT, P. H., GERBER, H. and MEISCHER, P. A. (1974). *J. clin. Invest.*, **54**, 297.

PEKIN, T. J. and ZVAIFLER, N. J. (1970). *Arthr. and Rheum.*, **13**, 777.

PERRIN, L. H., LAMBERT, P. H. and MIESCHER, P. A. (1975). *J. clin. Invest.*, **56**, 165.

PETZ, L. D., SHARP, G. C., COOPER, N. R. and IRVIN, W. S. (1971). *Medicine (Baltimore)*, **50**, 259.

PINCUS, T., BLACKLOW, N. R., GRIMLEY, P. M. and BELLANTI, J. A. (1970). *Lancet*, **2**, 1058.

POLLACK, V. E., PIRANI, C. L. (1974). In *Lupus Erythematosus*, 2nd edn., p. 73. Ed. E. L. Dubois. University of Southern California Press, Berkeley.

QUISMORIO, F. P. and FRIOU, G. J. (1972). *Int. Arch. Allergy appl. Immunol.*, **43**, 740.

SCHUR, P. H. and SANDSON, J. (1968). *New Engl. J. Med.*, **278**, 533.

SCHUR, P. H., STOLLAR, B. D., STEINBERG, A. D. and TALAL, N. (1971). *Arthr. and Rheum.*, **14**, 342.

SCHWARTZ, R. S. (1975). *New Engl. J. Med.*, **293**, 132.

SCHULMAN, N. R., MARDER, V. J. and WEINRACH, R. S. (1965). *Ann. N.Y. Acad. Sci.*, **124**, 499.

SWANSON BECK, J. and ROWELL, N. R. (1966). *Quart. J. Med.*, **35**, 119.

SYLVESTER, R. A., ATTIAS, M., TALAL, N. and TUFFANELLI, D. L. (1973). *Arthr. and Rheum.*, **16**, 383.

TAN, E. M. and KUNKEL, H. G. (1966). *Arthr. and Rheum.*, **9**, 37.

TANNENBAUM, H. and SCHUR, P. H. (1974). *J. Rheumatol.*, **1**, 392.

TERASAKI, P. I., MOTTIRONI, V. D. and BARNETT, E. V. (1970). *New Engl. J. Med.*, **283**, 724.

TUFFANELLI, D. L. and DUBOIS, E. L. (1964). *Arch. Derm.*, **90**, 377.

TUFFANELLI, D. L., KAY, D. and FUKUYAMA, K. (1969). *Arch. Derm.*, **99**, 652.

TURNER-WARWICK, M. (1974). *Proc. R. Soc. Med.*, **67**, 541.

UTERMOHLEN, V., WINFIELD, J. B. and KUNKEL, H. G. (1974). *J. exp. Med.*, **139**, 1019.

WILSON, C. B. and DIXON, F. J. (1971). *J. exp. med.*, **134**, 7.

WINCHESTER, R. J., WINFIELD, J. B., SIEGAL, E., WERNETT, P., BENTVICH, Z. and KUNKEL, H. G. (1974). *J. clin. Invest.*, **54**, 1082.

WINFIELD, J., KOFFLER, D. and KUNKEL, H. G. (1975). *J. clin. Invest.*, **56**, 563.
ZHDANOV, V. M. (1975). *Nature (Lond.)*, **256**, 471.
ZIFF, M. (1971). *Ann. intern. Med.*, 75, 951.
ZVEIMAN, B., KORNBIUM, J., CORNOG, J. and HILDRETH, E. A. (1968). *Ann. intern. Med.*,
    69, 441.

7

Sjögren's Syndrome

Clinical features

Sjögren's syndrome was described in 1933 and is characterized by diminished secretion of tears by the lacrimal gland and diminished production of saliva by the salivary gland. This leads to 'dry eyes' (xerophthalmia) and a 'dry mouth' (xerostomia). The xerophthalmia results in damage to the cornea and recurrent conjunctival inflammation, a syndrome described as keratoconjunctivitis sicca. The disease is characteristically seen in middle-aged women, and in about 50 per cent of such patients accompanies a polyarthritis resembling rheumatoid disease, or one of the other connective tissue diseases such as SLE or scleroderma. The classic triad of Sjögren's syndrome, therefore, comprises keratoconjunctivitis sicca, xerostomia and a connective tissue disease. (The combination of xerophthalmia and xerostomia alone is referred to as the 'sicca syndrome'.) Many patients with long-standing rheumatoid arthritis or antecedent systemic lupus erythematosus (or other connective tissue diseases) may also develop keratoconjunctivitis sicca and xerostomia, although the precise prevalence varies according to the criteria used for its diagnosis.

Biopsy of the affected lacrimal and salivary glands shows heavy infiltration of the tissue with mononuclear cells, both lymphocytes and plasma cells. A variable degree of atrophy and destruction of the acinar tissue is seen, replacing the normal lobular architecture. The lining cells of the salivary duct proliferate, giving rise to a characteristic microscopic appearance termed 'epimyoepithelial islands'.

Immunopathology

The technique of lower lip biopsy under local anaesthesia which enables examination of the minor salivary glands has been widely applied to study the tissue lesions in this disease. Fresh tissue sections obtained in this manner have been examined by immunofluorescent methods and shown to contain a large number of IgG-, IgM- and IgA-secreting plasma cells. The use of an anti-T-cell antiserum was used by Talal *et al.* (1974) to demonstrate T cells in the tissues, and these were found to be aggregated near the salivary ducts. Other workers employing EAC-rosette-forming techniques on fresh tissues have demonstrated aggregates of B cells in the parenchyma of the tissue (which accounted for a minority of cells) and were unable to show E-rosette-forming T cells, and concluded that the majority of lymphocytes could be null cells or T cells whose receptors were not available for E-rosette formation (Tannenbaum *et al.*, 1975). Whether the T cells are functioning as helper cells or have a more direct role in producing tissue injury remains problematical, the difficulty in assessing their significance being similar to the findings in rheumatoid synovial tissue (see Chapter 5, on rheumatoid arthritis).

Another similarity of salivary gland inflammation to rheumatoid synovitis is the demonstration by Anderson *et al.* (1972) of immunoglobulin synthesis by cultures of explants of lip biopsies. All classes of immunoglobulin appear to be synthesized in organ cultures established from patients with Sjögren's syndrome but, in contrast to cultures from control subjects, greatly increased amounts of IgM and IgG are synthesized. The control cultures, however, synthesized matching levels of IgA—the immunoglobulin normally secreted in the saliva. In these studies it was also shown that the supernatants of the organ cultures contained rheumatoid factor activity, thus demonstrating the nature of one of the antibodies being synthesized in the salivary gland. The local synthesis of immunoglobulin, especially with rheumatoid factor activity, also bears resemblance to the secretion of rheumatoid synovial tissue.

Autoantibodies

A number of autoantibodies appear to be frequently present in the sera of patients with Sjögren's syndrome. These include:

1. In one series (Bunim *et al.*, 1964) almost every patient studied had detectable rheumatoid factor in the serum. In other studies the proportion of patients with such antibodies was in the region of 60–80 per cent. The levels of rheumatoid factor tend to be extremely high, and occur irrespective of whether co-existing rheumatoid arthritis is present or not.

2. Anti-nuclear factors have been detected in 50–60 per cent of patients with Sjögren's syndrome. A homogeneous pattern of nuclear immunofluorescence is usually observed, but some workers (Beck *et al.*, 1964) have commented on the observation that a significant proportion of sera from patients showed a speckled pattern. Using well characterized antigens, it has been possible to demonstrate antibodies to both single- and double-stranded DNA, and at least in one study, antibodies to extractable nuclear antigens were also present.

3. The prevalence of autoantibodies to salivary duct cells has been demonstrated by a number of workers. These autoantibodies stain the cytoplasm of the duct epithelial cells and are demonstrated by an immunofluorescent technique. Their prevalence in separate studies carried out in Glasgow and at the National Institute of Health in Bethesda was 10–20 per cent in patients with keratoconjunctivitis sicca alone and up to 70 per cent in patients with Sjögren's syndrome with rheumatoid arthritis (reviewed by Cummings *et al.*, 1971). Patients

with rheumatoid arthritis without Sjögren's syndrome also showed the antibody in up to 40 per cent of sera. The significance of this antibody remains an enigma. Its finding in patients with rheumatoid arthritis and other connective tissue diseases without Sjögren's syndrome would seem to indicate that it is not of pathogenetic importance in the pathogenesis of salivary gland lesions. It also does not appear to have the same clinical significance as organ-specific antibodies occurring in diseases such as autoimmune thyroiditis, Addison's disease and pernicious anaemia.

4. The prevalence of antibodies to other antigens (e.g. smooth muscle, mitochondria, gastric parietal cells and thyroid antigens) is variable in published studies, with an over-all suggestion of an increased incidence in the Sjögren's syndrome group. In another study on Sjögren's syndrome, however (Feltkamp and van Rossum, 1968), there was an increase in the prevalence of rheumatoid factor, anti-nuclear, anti-salivary-gland and smooth muscle antibody, but not of antibody to mitochondria, gastric parietal cells or thyroid antigens when compared with matched controls.

Cell-mediated immunity

LYMPHOCYTE FUNCTION

Studies of lymphocyte function in Sjögren's syndrome have generally shown a depression of various parameters of cellular hypersensitivity. Thus, skin tests to various antigens (e.g. PPD) have been shown to be depressed; sensitization to DNCB has shown a decreased level of reaction, and lymphocyte transformation tests with antigen and mitogens a depressed response. These results are much more consistent than comparable findings in patients with rheumatoid arthritis (see Chapter 5).

ENUMERATION OF PERIPHERAL LYMPHOCYTE POPULATIONS

Results of studies of the composition of populations of peripheral blood lymphocytes in Sjögren's syndrome suggest that there may usually be an increase in B cells, and that in some patients a decrease in T cells may occur (Talal *et al.*, 1974). In a study in which the heavy chain specificity of the surface immunoglobulin on B cells was enumerated, it was found that cells bearing at least two of these heavy chain markers were elevated compared to controls (van Boxel *et al.*, 1973). This finding indicated that individual B cells in some patients with Sjögren's syndrome bear multiple classes of heavy chain, a finding which resembled the abnormality noted by other workers in patients with lymphoproliferative disease.

The finding of reduced numbers of T cells in peripheral blood in Sjögren's syndrome is of possible relevance to the observed findings of depressed cellular immunity. From the functional point of view the depressed cellular immunity in these patients has been regarded as being a significant factor in loss of surveillance function of cellular immunity, which leads to the increased prevalence of lymphomas.

Relationship to lymphoproliferative disorders

Patients with Sjögren's syndrome show an apparently increased tendency to develop lymphoreticular malignancy and pseudo-lymphoma (reviewed by Anderson and Talal, 1971). This is characterized clinically by the development of lymphadenopathy, hepatosplenomegaly and, in some patients, an IgM monoclonal para-proteinaemia. Lymphadenopathy by itself is not an unusual finding in patients with autoimmune disease; for example, in rheumatoid arthritis and SLE. However, lymph node biopsies in patients with rheumatoid arthritis usually show a follicular hyperplasia, the appearance indicating local antigenic stimulation. In contrast to this, lymph nodes of patients with Sjögren's syndrome show not only enlargement but also a pleomorphic infiltrate of cells with frequent mitosis, penetration of the capsule and obscuring of the sinuses. An increased number of normal lymphoid cells (i.e. lymphocytes and plasma cells), reticulum cells as well as primitive cells are seen in the lymph nodes. Some of these cells appear to be locally invasive, penetrating the capsule and the adjacent connective tissue; several of the cells appear to have large nucleioli, little cytoplasm and contain PAS-positive material in the nucleus. This appearance has been described as 'pseudo-lymphoma', since the full criteria for a malignant lymphoma are not satisfied. However, several patients have been described in whom a frank reticulum cell sarcoma was observed and led to a fatal outcome (Talal *et al.*, 1967).

IgM para-proteinaemia in Sjögren's syndrome has been well documented in several cases. It is of interest that many patients with Sjögren's syndrome, especially those developing pseudo-lymphoma or a genuine lymphoma, may show an increased level of IgM protein of a polyclonal nature. The synthesis of IgM immunoglobulin by the salivary gland may be of relevance to this finding.

The features of Sjögren's syndrome described above have led Talal to observe that the disorder lies 'somewhere between hyperplasia and neoplasia' and, in his view, genetic, viral and environmental factors might be operating together to produce the disease syndrome. Attention has been drawn by Talal to the similarity of salivary gland infiltrate observed in New Zealand mice who are susceptible to autoimmune diseases (see Cummings *et al.*, 1971). The possible role of virus induction of Sjögren's syndrome has been suggested by the presence of virus-like tubular structures in renal biopsies from patients with renal interstitial and tubular disorders sometimes seen in the syndrome (see Chapter 6).

References

ANDERSON, L. G. and TALAL, N. (1971). *Clin. exp. Immunol.*, **9**, 199.

ANDERSON, L. G., CUMMINGS, N. A., ASOFSKY, R., HYLTON, M. B., TARPLEY, T. M., TOMASI, T. S., WOLF, R. O., SCHALL, G. L. and TALAL, N. (1972). *Amer. J. Med.*, **53**, 546.

BECK, J. S., ANDERSON, J. R., BLOCH, K. J., BUCHANAN, W. W. and BUNIM, J. J. (1964). *Ann. rheum. Dis.*, **24**, 16.

BUNIM, J. J., BUCHANAN, W. W., WERTLAKE, P. T., SOKOLOFF, L., BLOCH, K. J., BECK, J. W. and ALEPA, F. P. (1964). *Ann. intern. Med.*, **61**, 509.

CUMMINGS, N. A., SCHALL, G. L., ASOFSKY, R., ANDERSON, L. G. and TALAL, N. (1971). *Ann. intern. Med.*, **75**, 937.

FELTKAMP, T. E. W., VAN ROSSUM, A. L. (1968). *Clin. exp. Immunol.*, **3**, 1.

TALAL, N., SOKOLOFF, L. and BARTH, W. F. (1967). *Amer. J. Med.*, **43**, 50.

TALAL, N., SYLVESTER, R. A., DANIELS, T. E., GREENSPAN, J. S. and WILLIAMS, R. C. (1974). *J. clin. Invest.*, **53**, 180.

TANNENBAUM, H., PINKUS, G. S., ANDERSON, L. G. and SCHUR, P. H. (1975). *Arthr. and Rheum.* **18**, 30.

VAN BOXEL, J. A., HARDIN, J. A., GREEN, I. and PAUL, W. E. (1973). *New Engl. J. Med.*, **289**, 823.

8

Polymyositis and Myasthenia Gravis

Introduction

Polymyositis and myasthenia gravis are amongst the diseases of muscle which exhibit a number of immunological abnormalities, some of which appear to be related to their pathogenesis. In certain 'inflammatory' vascular diseases muscles are involved (e.g. polyarteritis nodosa) and immunological processes are implicated, but the primary disorder is demonstrably vascular, and is discussed in Chapter 11. In diseases such as rheumatoid arthritis and systemic lupus erythematosus, muscle pains, tenderness and wasting are not uncommon, but in the presence of disease of adjacent joints the symptoms may result from referred pain arising from shared spinal segmental innervation of joints and muscles, and wasting may result from disuse. Histological examination of muscles in these diseases may show lymphocyte infiltration of doubtful pathological significance, and it is arguable whether a primary muscle disorder exists. However, a more florid polymyositis can occur in association with connective tissue diseases. Myasthenia gravis associated with thyrotoxicosis is well recognized and is sometimes seen with other autoimmune diseases. It has recently been recognized as a reversible complication during the use of the drug D-penicillamine in the treatment of rheumatoid arthritis and Wilson's disease (a disease of abnormal metabolism of copper). Corticosteroid drugs and chloroquine, both used in the treatment of connective tissue diseases, may also cause a myopathy.

Clinicopathological features

Polymyositis has been classified in a variety of ways. That recommended by the International Research Group on neuromuscular disorders suggests three main types (Walton, 1968): α, β and γ.

1. TYPE α

This is 'uncomplicated' polymyositis, involving muscles without any obvious skin involvement, and with no associated or underlying disease.

2. TYPE β

Type β is seen as dermatomyositis or in association with a connective tissue disease. The typical skin involvement of dermatomyositis appears as an erythematous, slightly scaly, rash on the hands, fingers and elbows, and is accompanied by a heliotrope discoloration of the upper eyelids. The connective tissue diseases with which polymyositis occurs most frequently are Sjögren's syndrome, scleroderma, systemic lupus erythematosus, rheumatoid arthritis, and the less well defined 'mixed connective tissue disease'.

3. TYPE γ

Type γ polymyositis (or dermatomyositis) is associated with a neoplasm (of bronchus, breast, prostate, ovary, uterus or large intestine).

Myasthenia gravis, which is characterized by muscle weakness and fatiguability with a typical abnormality of neuromuscular transmission, is regarded as clinically and pathophysiologically distinct from polymyositis. On closer inspection, however, some similarities between the two conditions are seen and they may co-exist.

The distribution of weakness of muscles may be generalized in both conditions and produce a superficially identical clinical picture. Involvement of certain localized muscle groups is, however, more characteristic of polymyositis; for example, limb-girdle, proximal and axial muscle involvement (although this distribution is not specific as it is also seen in other diseases, for example, in Cushing's syndrome, and thyrotoxicosis). Involvement of extraocular and facial muscles, on the other hand, causing double vision and ptosis are more typical of myasthenia gravis. Pain and tenderness of muscles are not marked but may be present in polymyositis. Progressive fatiguability on repeated or sustained contraction of muscles is of course usual in myasthenia gravis, with a dramatic and instantaneous recovery following administration of anticholinesterase inhibitors (but cases resistant to this treatment are recognized). Electromyographic studies in myasthenia gravis are diagnostic of the condition if, on stimulation of nerves or on active contraction of muscle, they show a diminished amplitude of successive muscle potentials. This abnormality is reversed with anticholinesterase inhibitors. In polymyositis, electromyography shows a variety of non-specific changes suggestive of muscle damage. Thymic dysplasia or neoplasia is usual in myasthenia gravis and may be accompanied by an enlargement of the thymus gland, the latter finding being of diagnostic value. In contrast, polymyositis may co-exist with neoplasms of bronchus, etc.

Damage of muscle fibres and an inflammatory response are essential features of polymyositis. Fragmentation and necrosis of muscle fibres is seen, and the infiltrating mononuclear cells (lymphocytes and plasma cells) are sometimes observed to be in contact with the muscle membrane, so as to suggest a direct cytotoxic effect. Perivascular infiltration of cells, however, is also usual, and is seen most obviously in the peri-myesial veins. Interstitial infiltrates of mononuclear cells are also common. Fibre damage, however, to a certain extent, is also apparent in certain patients with myasthenia gravis (reviewed by Irvine and

Kalden, 1975) as is cellular infiltration of the interstitium but it is difficult to rule out an associated 'polymyositis'. In one reported study (Whitaker and Engel, 1972) a 'vasculitic' process was thought to be present especially in muscle biopsies of children with dermatomyositis, raising the possibility that in these cases muscle damage was secondary to vascular occlusion (see below). As might be expected, raised levels of muscle enzymes, such as creatinine phosphokinase, are a constant feature of polymyositis.

The similarity in clinicopathological features in these two conditions may reflect the limited expression of changes possible in any damaged tissue, and in this respect are probably 'non-specific'. Other changes sometimes observed in muscle biopsies (for example, accumulation of a small number of mononuclear lymphocytes) also occur in control populations and appear to be of trivial or doubtful significance. A more serious problem arises in distinguishing between changes which primarily mediate tissue injury, from those that are consequent upon the injury. In assessing muscle pathology account must also be taken of changes (especially those leading to fibre atrophy) secondary to disuse of muscles as a consequence of prolonged bed-rest or lack of movement due to pain in adjacent joints, and possible effects of drugs such as steroids.

Furthermore, although usually considered as single entities, each of the two disorders (polymyositis and myasthenia gravis) represents a heterogeneous group of conditions in terms of variability and extent of clinical and pathological involvement, immunological abnormalities, and environmental and genetic factors thought to be involved in aetiology.

Immunology of polymyositis

Autoimmune humoral and cellular pathogenetic mechanisms, as well as immune complex involvement, have been sought in polymyositis. To date, evidence of cellular mechanisms has been forthcoming in human polymyositis, with little convincing evidence of antibody-mediated damage. The following studies are noted:

Autoantibodies

Caspary and his colleagues (1964) showed an increased incidence of anti-nuclear factors in patients with polymyositis although their occurrence may have reflected the associated connective tissue disease in some patients. Anti-skeletal-muscle antibodies in serum can be demonstrated using muscle antigens in techniques such as agglutination of tanned red blood cells, complement fixation and gel-diffusion precipitation, or employing sections of muscle tissue in immuno-fluorescent studies. However, in published studies, significant differences have rarely been demonstrated between patients with polymyositis and controls (Caspary *et al.*, 1964; Fessel and Raas, 1968).

Immune complexes

In a study of 39 patients with idiopathic polymyositis (Whitaker and Engel, 1972), 17 patients showed deposits of IgG, IgM together with C3 alone or in combination in skeletal-muscle blood vessels (usually peri-myesial veins). The authors of this study remarked on the especially high prevalence of this abnormality in childhood dermatomyositis, and commented that most of the vessels containing deposits appeared to be either normal on light microscopy, or showed minimal thickening of intima. In the same study deposition of immunoglobulin and C3 in structurally abnormal muscle fibres was found in a variety of diseases used as controls and was not thought to be specific for polymyositis. It is surprising that a role for immune-complex-mediated tissue damage has not been shown in patients with polymyositis associated with connective tissue diseases such as SLE in which complexes in other organs have been demonstrated.

Cellular hypersensitivity

Evidence of circulating lymphocytes sensitized to muscle antigen has been obtained in a number of studies. Using lymphocyte transformation tests, Currie and his colleagues (1971) showed stimulation of thymidine incorporation in lymphocytes cultured with muscle homogenates. The same group were also able to demonstrate lymphocyte-mediated cytotoxicity using peripheral lymphocytes from patients with polymyositis cultured with human fetal muscle cultures. The findings were extended by Johnson *et al.* (1972), who also showed the participation of the lymphokine mediator, lymphotoxin, in such toxic reactions. These findings have been confirmed by others (see Dawkins and Dilko, 1975).

Experimental models

Injection of muscle homogenates in Freund's adjuvant leads to the production of a polymyositis in guinea-pigs or rats. The lymphocytes from these animals are cytotoxic to muscle cultures *in vitro* (Kakulas, 1966), and are capable of transferring the disease to healthy recipients in cell transfer experiments (for references see Currie *et al.*, 1971). These animals also develop delayed hypersensitivity reactions and give positive lymphocyte transformation tests with muscle antigens. These results indicate the participation of T cell reactions. In the experimental model in guinea-pigs (unlike the human disease) evidence has also been produced to demonstrate the frequent occurrence of skeletal muscle antibodies using a variety of techniques (reviewed by Dawkins and Dilko, 1975). It could be suggested that by opsonizing muscle, such antibodies facilitate interaction with K cells, mononuclear phagocytes or neutrophils, and damage muscle (Chapter 2).

ASSOCIATION WITH IMMUNODEFICIENCY AND NEOPLASTIC DISEASE

The observations that polymyositis may occur in some patients with hypogammaglobulinaemia and that patients with polymyositis show diminished secondary antibody responses, led Dawkins and Dilko (1975) to speculate that humoral deficiency may be an important predisposing factor in the development of a T-cell mediated reaction. It was suggested that the association with neo-plastic disease may be similarly explained on the basis of a general humoral deficiency. This idea leaves unanswered the clinical observation that removal of neoplastic tissue may be accompanied by remission of polymyositis, and that, in the generally accepted view, T cell immune surveillance (rather than humoral immunity) is of central importance. The possibility that the neoplastic tissue actively induces autoimmunity (e.g. by antigen cross-reaction with muscle) requires consideration (see Chapter 1, section on 'Cellular mechanisms of auto-immunity').

Immunology of myasthenia gravis

The nature of the lesion which leads to defective neuromuscular transmission at the motor end-plate in myasthenia gravis, potentially reversible with the use of anticholinesterase drugs, remains ill understood. It is not certain whether the defect is pre-synaptic (i.e. involved with the synthesis or secretion of acetyl-choline) or post-synaptic (i.e. a fault in the receptor at the motor end-plate). Studies have shown a diminution in the number of motor end-plates in myas-thenia gravis and, more recently, it has been suggested that autoantibodies to the end-plate receptor may functionally interfere with transmission of nerve impulses (see below). The association, especially in young females, with HL-A-8 (Felt-kamp *et al.*, 1974) raises the possibility of genetic susceptibility, and induction of myasthenia gravis in those receiving D-penicillamine for rheumatoid arthritis, which reverses on cessation of the drug, presumably provides a clue to the environmental trigger in this disease.

THYMUS AND ANTI-SKELETAL MUSCLE ANTIBODIES

The frequently observed changes in the thymus gland in patients with myas-thenia have attracted a great deal of attention. In about 10 per cent of patients, tumours of the thymus gland are present, whereas in the rest, the gland may be of normal size or slightly enlarged but usually shows histological abnormalities. These changes include the prominent formation of lymphoid follicles with germinal centres, with an increased number of mononuclear cells and presence of myoid cells (the latter cells resembling skeletal muscle cells, and normally only found in fetal thymic tissue). These histological changes, however, are not specific but are possibly suggestive of antigen stimulation.

The sera of patients with myasthenia gravis frequently contain an antibody to skeletal muscle which cross-reacts with thymic epithelial cells, believed to be derived from myoid cells (reviewed by Irvine and Kalden, 1975). In fact the anti-skeletal muscle antibodies are heterogeneous in terms of class, complement-fixing ability, antigenic specificity and their cross-reactivity with thymic tissue. Such antibodies are present, especially in patients with severe disease of recent onset (as many as 68 per cent of patients showing this antibody by immuno-fluorescence in a study by Osserman and Weiner, 1965). A correlation of the antibody with thymomas (with or without myasthenia gravis) has also been noted. Doubts have been expressed about the pathogenicity of the autoantibody since these antibodies may be found in patients without myasthenia gravis (including control groups as well as children born to mothers with myasthenia acquiring antibody via placental transfer); and, conversely, because several patients with the myasthenia syndrome do not have antibodies. It has not been possible to demonstrate localization of anti-muscle antibodies in the motor end-plate. In patients with anti-skeletal muscle antibody, Dawkins and Dilko (1975) noted that lymphocyte-mediated cytotoxicity of muscle *in vitro* was as pronounced as that observed in polymyositis.

ANTI-NUCLEAR, LYMPHOCYTOTOXIC AND ANTI-RECEPTOR ANTIBODIES

Other antibodies which have been found in myasthenia gravis include anti-nuclear factor found in up to 30 per cent of patients and thyroid antibodies in approximately 40 per cent of patients.

Lymphocytotoxins reactive at 15°C have also been found in a significant number of patients with myasthenia gravis (for references see Irvine and Kalden, 1975), a result reminiscent of the findings in connective tissue disease such as systemic lupus erythematosus and rheumatoid arthritis.

Of considerable interest is the finding of an antibody to the motor end-plate receptor. The possibility that receptor antibodies may be involved in the pathogenesis of myasthenia gravis was suggested by the experiments of Patrick and Linstrom (1973) who showed that motor end-plate receptors extracted from the electric eel when injected into rabbits led to an immune response which coincided with the development of a myasthenia-type illness. *In vitro* experiments have shown that α-bungarotoxin (extracted from snake venom) has a high affinity for the motor end-plate receptors and compete with a globulin in the serum of patients with myasthenia gravis. A recently developed radioimmunoassay employing radioisotopically labelled α-bungarotoxin complexed to extracted motor end-plate has shown the presence of antibody to receptors in the sera of the majority of patients with myasthenia gravis (Appel *et al.*, 1975). These experiments have led to the attractive hypothesis that myasthenia gravis may, in a large number of patients, result from interference with receptor function mediated by an antibody. The relationship of such an antibody to previously demonstrated anti-skeletal muscle antibody remains to be elucidated.

THYMIC FACTORS

The possibility that the thymus might generate a circulating factor which interferes with neuromuscular junction transmission was based partly on the observation that thymectomy is of therapeutic value in myasthenia gravis. A polypeptide extracted from calf thymus (termed 'thymin') causes neuromuscular block of the type seen in myasthenia when injected into rats and guinea-pigs (Goldstein and Manganaro, 1971). The physiological role of thymin and its relationship to a factor present in human blood and termed 'thymic hormone' is uncertain. Bach and his associates (1972) detected thymic hormone (also a peptide) by its ability to restore the blocking effects of anti-thymocyte serum or azathioprine on the ability of spleen cells from adult thymectomized mice to form rosettes with sheep erythrocytes. These workers have found that thymic hormone serum levels are high in normal children and decrease with age in adults. In patients in whom thymectomy was performed for myasthenia gravis, the level fell to undetectable amounts within 24 hours. Whilst it is uncertain whether thymic hormone is of clinical significance in myasthenia gravis, its levels in patients with SLE have been found to be lower than in controls, and higher in rheumatoid arthritis (Bach *et al.*, 1975). It has been suggested that thymic hormone might play a part in controlling T lymphocyte function.

CELLULAR IMMUNITY

Alpert *et al.* (1972) have reported that, using crude muscle extract and the muscle protein, actomyosin, as an antigen, leucocyte migration in a capillary tube method was inhibited in a significant proportion of patients with myasthenia gravis. The finding of increased toxicity to muscle *in vitro* by lymphocytes from patients with myasthenia gravis further suggested a role for cellular immunity.

The relative importance of and the inter-relationships between these cellular observations and the abnormalities of humoral immunity require further elucidation, as does the apparent relationship of myasthenia gravis to polymyositis.

References

ALPERT, L. I., RULE, A., NORIO, M., KOTT, E., KORNFELD, P. and OSSERMAN, K. E. (1972). *Amer. J. clin. Path.*, **58**, 647.

APPEL, S. H., ALMON, R. R. and LEVY, N. (1975). *New Engl. J. Med.*, **293**, 760.

BACH, J. F., DARDENNE, M., PAPIERNIK, M., BAROIS, A., LEVASSEUR, M. and LEBRIGAND, H. (1972). *Lancet*, **2**, 1056.

BACH, J. F., DARDENNE, M. and CLOT, J. (1975). *Rheumatology*, **6**, 242.

CASPARY, E. A., GUBAY, S. S. and STERN, G. M. (1964). *Lancet*, **2**, 941.

CURRIE, S., SAUNDERS, M., KNOWLES, M. and BROWN, A. E. (1971). *Quart. J. Med.* (*N.S.*), **157**, 63.

DAWKINS, R. L. and DILKO, P. J. (1975). *Lancet*, **1**, 200.

FELTKAMP, T. E. W., VAN DEN BERG-LOONEN, NIJENHUIS, L. E., ENLEFRIET, C. P., VAN ROSSUM, A. L., VANLOGHEM, J. J. and OOSTERHUIS, H. J. G. (1974). *Brit. med. J.*, **1**, 131.

FESSEL, W. J. and RAAS, M. C. (1968). *Neurology (Minneap.)*, **18**, 1137.

GOLDSTEIN, G. and MANGANARO, A. (1971), *Ann. N.Y. Acad. Sci.*, **183**, 230.

IRVINE, W. J. and KALDEN, J. R. (1975). In *Clinical Aspects of Immunology*, p. 1467. Ed. P. G. H. Gell, R. R. A. Coombs and P. J. Lachmann. Blackwell Scientific Publications, Oxford.

JOHNSON, R. L., FINK, C. W. and ZIFF, M. (1972). *J. clin. Invest.*, **51**, 2435.

KAKULAS, B. A. (1966). *Nature (Lond.)*, **210**, 1165.

OSSERMAN, K. E. and WEINER, L. B. (1965). *New Engl. J. Med.* **273**, 615.

PATRICK, J. and LINSTROM, J. (1973). *Science*, **180**, 871.

WALTON, J. N. (1968). *J. neurol. Sci.*, **6**, 165.

WHITAKER, J. N. and ENGEL, W. K. (1972). *New Engl. J. Med.*, **286**, 333.

9

Relapsing Polychondritis

Relapsing polychondritis, although rare, provides a possible example of a disease which may be mediated by immune reactions directed against specific antigens present in connective tissue matrix. The clinical features of the condition have been reviewed by Dolan *et al.* (1966); it is characterized by destruction of hyaline cartilage of the ears, nose and the rings of the trachea and bronchi, and, less commonly, articular cartilage. Histological examination of the area of junction between cartilage and loose connective tissue during periods of acute inflammation, shows infiltration with plasma cells, lymphocytes and polymorphs. The possibility that tissue damage may be mediated by immune complexes or a local Arthus type hypersensitivity was suggested by the finding of serum antibodies against cartilage components in these patients, but low titres of antibodies were also found in patients with rheumatoid arthritis (Hughes *et al.*, 1972). In several other studies, however, antibodies to articular cartilage of individual matrix components, for example proteoglycans, were not demonstrated (reviewed by Rajapakse and Bywaters, 1974).

Lymphocyte transformation with crude antigen extracts prepared from cartilage and chondrocyte fractions was observed to be positive in patients with polychondritis, but doubts about the specificity of these results were raised because rheumatoid arthritis patients also showed a positive response (Herman and Dennis, 1973). In another study in which biochemically defined proteoglycan was used as an antigen, more clear-cut evidence of cellular immunity appeared to be obtained and was found to be confined to patients with relapsing polychondritis (Rajapakse and Bywaters, 1974). In this study, inhibition of migration of guinea-pig peritoneal macrophages mixed with human lymphocytes was used as an indicator of cellular hypersensitivity. Two patients with Takayasu's disease ('pulseless syndrome'), one of whom also suffered from chondritis, have been reported to have shown positive results in the same *in vitro* test (Rajapakse and Bywaters, 1973). On this basis it has been suggested that cell-mediated reactions to proteoglycan antigens (present in cartilage and arterial wall) may be of pathogenetic significance.

References

DOLAN, D. L., LEMMON, G. B. and TEITELBAUM, S. L. (1966). *Amer. J. Med.*, **41**, 285.

HERMAN, J. H. and DENNIS, M. V. (1973). *J. clin. Invest.*, **52**, 549.

HUGHES, R. A. C., BERRY, C. L., SIEFERT, M. and LESSOF, M. H. (1972). *Quart. J. Med. (N.S.)*, **163**, 363.

RAJAPAKSE, D. A. and BYWATERS, E. G. L. (1973), *Brit. med. J.*, **4**, 488.

RAJAPAKSE, D. A. and BYWATERS, E. G. L. (1974). *Clin. exp. Immunol.*, **16**, 497.

10

Infections and Arthritis

Introduction

The occurrence of arthritis in association with known infectious agents provides an insight into the nature of immunopathogenetic mechanisms involved in producing arthritis on the one hand, and an understanding of host–microbial relationships on the other. It also provides an important opportunity for a better understanding of the pathogenesis of diseases in which an infectious aetiology is very likely but not yet proven, such as Reiter's disease, as well as diseases such as rheumatoid arthritis and systemic lupus erythematosus for which an infective aetiology is proposed but remains largely speculative.

Non-specific symptoms referred to the musculoskeletal system, as well as myalgias and arthralgias, are not unusual in infectious diseases. Certain infections, however, are associated with an observable arthritis occurring during the course of infection, either in the prodromal period or in the stage of the established infection, or some days after the infection has apparently subsided. The clinical features of the arthritis are diverse; for example, the arthritis may affect a single joint (monarthritis), two or three joints (oligoarthritis) or several joints (polyarthritis). The arthritis may be 'flitting' in character as seen in rheumatic fever, or appear as an established arthritis with signs of acute or chronic inflammation. Tendon sheaths may also be involved. Joint effusions may occur, and their composition may be that of a purulent exudate, or an exudate containing greater or lesser numbers of polymorphs or lymphocytes. Large mononuclear cells in synovial fluid have been found in arthritis occurring in viral diseases.

Some of the organisms which are associated with an arthritis are shown in Table 10.1. These include: bacteria, with either cocciform (a to e) or bacilliform (f to k) morphology; viruses whose core is composed of ribonucleic acid (l to n) and deoxyribonucleic acid (o to q) and other organisms such as Chlamydia which belong to the psitticosis–lymphogranulomatrachoma group (r); or fungi such as coccidioidomycosis (s). Clinical experience shows that demonstration of the organism by microscopy or its isolation by culture is easily performed in the case of certain organisms, whereas other organisms are rarely, if ever, found. The lack of demonstration of an organism can result from a variety of causes; for example, it may merely reflect unsuitable or inadequate isolation techniques (as

Table 10.1   Some infectious agents associated with an arthritis

Bacteria	*Viruses*
a. Staphylococci	l. Rubella
b. Streptococci	m. Mumps
c. Pneumococci	n. Arboviruses
d. Gonococci	o. Hepatitis B virus
e. Meningococci	(Australia antigen)
	p. Infectious mononucleosis
f. Salmonella	(Ebstein–Barr virus)
g. Shigella	q. Smallpox
h. *Yersinia Enterocolitica*	
i. Brucella	*Others*
j. *Mycobacterium tuberculosis*	r. Chlamydia
k. *Mycobacterium leprosae*	s. Coccidioidomycosis

in the case of certain viruses), transient presence of the organism in the joint, its inhibition or neutralization by factors present in the joint fluid, or prior antibiotic therapy. In other instances in which an immune pathogenesis may be implicated, the organisms may not be present in a viable form, but may still provide immunogenic material. The presence in joint fluids of such microbial antigens would be of equal interest, but these are not often sought. Indeed a systematic and full microbiological and immunological documentation in arthritis occurring in association with most forms of infection is sadly lacking.

Classification

It is possible to suggest a classification of arthritis associated with infections based on whether or not the organism (or antigens derived from it) localize in the joint, and whether or not immune response contributes significantly to the pathogenesis. However, it has to be conceded that this approach is at present limited, owing to lack of adequate data. Four categories may be recognized:

1. Arthritis in which the infectious agent, having found access to the joint, multiplies locally and does not elicit any significant specific immunological reactivity.

In such forms of arthritis the organism is readily demonstrated in the synovial fluid and membrane and signs of sepsis are apparent. Organisms which can cause this type of 'septic arthritis' include bacteria (e.g. staphylococci, pneumococci and gonococci), viruses (e.g. smallpox and varicella) and certain fungi (e.g. coccidioidomycosis). Although such infections may arise in apparently healthy individuals, they are more liable to occur in previously diseased joints (for example, rheumatoid joints) or in patients whose protective immune responses are compromised (for example, those suffering from reticulosis, immunodeficiency or patients receiving large doses of steroids).

2. Arthritis in which the infectious agents (or antigens derived from it) localize in the joint and are associated with an immune response relevant to the pathogenesis of arthritis. Several types of immunological reactions could be envisaged. For example:

(a) The organism (or its antigen) may, in an immunized host, give rise to local type III or type IV hypersensitivity reactions. The role of such mechanisms in naturally occurring infectious arthritis is largely unevaluated, but is better recognized in certain forms of experimental arthritis. In swine, intraperitoneal innoculation of *Mycoplasma hyorhinis* produces a chronic arthritis closely resembling rheumatoid disease. In the first few months the organisms can be cultured from blood and joint tissues, but later isolation proves to be impossible. At this later stage mycoplasma antigens can, however, be demonstrated in the synovium by employing antisera in immunofluorescent techniques, as can local antibody synthesis (Decker and Barden, 1975). These findings, together with the demonstration of delayed hypersensitivity reactions to Mycoplasma antigen (accompanied by a flare-up of the arthritis), suggest that type III and type IV reactions occur in the joint. In another model, injection of herpes simplex virus in the joints of rabbits and guinea-pigs results in a chronic synovitis accompanied by acquisition of cellular immunity although persistence of virus cannot be demonstrated (Bacon *et al.*, 1974). The arthritis seen in patients suffering from rubella, which occasionally persists for a few weeks and in which virus from joints has been isolated, might be an example of a similar naturally occurring disease. It is tempting to suggest similar mechanisms in rheumatoid disease to, as yet, undefined organisms.

(b) The arthritis might occur as a result of deposition of circulating immune complexes in joints. This mechanism has been suspected in certain forms of hepatitis B infection and meningococcal arthritis (see below).

3. Arthritis in which the infectious agent is located at a distant site from the joint, but in which immune mechanisms are believed to play an important part. Examples include:

(a) Infection by an organism distant from the joint, and often preceding the onset of arthritis which, by virtue of antigens which cross-react with host antigens, sets in train the development of autoantibodies which are associated with a disease process; e.g. streptococcal throat infection and rheumatic fever (see below).

(b) Arthritis following infection by an organism in which the participation of immune mechanisms is suspected but not yet documented or elucidated are included in this category. Gastrointestinal infections with Shigella and Salmonella have long been recognized to precede one type of Reiter's disease. More recently, gastrointestinal infection with *Yersinia enterocolitica*, a gram-negative organism, has also been recognized to give rise to a 'reactive' polyarthritis. In these groups of patients a very high incidence of HL-A-27 tissue serotype has been found (Aho *et al.*, 1975), thus linking the phenotype with susceptibility to an inflammatory polyarthritis associated with an infection. The strong association between HL-A-27 and Reiter's disease acquires added significance when viewed against this background as, in this case, arthritis follows an apparently non-specific urethritis which is nevertheless known to be of infectious aetiology on epidemiological grounds.

4. Arthritis (or arthralgias) may occur during the height of infections, in which case it is unlikely that immune mechanisms are involved. This type of

symptom may result from arthritogenic toxic products of viruses or bacteria; for example, in epidemic forms of arbovirus infections (Smith and Sanford, 1967).

An important limitation of this classification is the possibility that any single organism may cause an arthritis due to more than one type of mechanism. For example, in certain patients with meningococcal infection the organism may be isolated from the joints, whereas in the majority it is not. Conversely, in certain patients with proven gonococcal infections, a hypersensitivity type of arthritis has been suspected since an arthritis has been observed to follow effective elimination of the organisms by antibiotics, although, in such cases, coincidental occurrence of Reiter's syndrome associated with a non-specific urethritis is difficult to exclude. In patients with rubella, too, more than one type of mechanism might operate, since arthritis may sometimes develop in the prodromal period, whilst in others it can occur at the height of the exanthematous rash, or follow recovery. Its duration also varies from a few days to a few weeks and, in the latter instance, the picture may clinically resemble rheumatoid arthritis, although the arthritis (with the exception of one recorded instance) invariably resolves.

In the classification presented here, much emphasis has been placed on specific microbial immunity. However, it has been recognized that many infections are accompanied by the appearance of autoantibodies—for example, rheumatoid factor and anti-nuclear factor occur in leprosy; rheumatoid factor in subacute bacterial endocarditis, rubella, infectious mononucleosis and viral pneumonia; anti-nuclear factors and smooth muscle antibody in a number of viral infections, as well as parasitic infections. Their possible role in initiating an arthritis and mediating tissue lesions is very uncertain although it is of interest that in some of these diseases a polyarthritis resembling rheumatoid arthritis is seen, for example in leprosy and rubella. The possibility that these autoantibodies circulate as immune complexes is supported by the findings of cryoglobulins in some of these infections. In a few instances, immune complex nephritis may also occur; for example, in infectious mononucleosis and subacute bacterial endocarditis. In the laboratory models of viral immune complex nephritis in mice (e.g. lymphocytic choriomeningitis virus infection) anti-nuclear antibodies and antigens have been shown to contribute significantly to the immune complex deposits in kidneys (see Chapter 6).

Rheumatic fever

It is accepted that rheumatic fever arises as a consequence of immunological reactions following infection with any one of 50 or more types of group A haemolytic streptococci, a subject fully and admirably reviewed by Glynn (1975). This view has been substantiated by epidemiological studies in which attacks of rheumatic fever were found to follow in up to 3 per cent of patients with bacteriologically confirmed upper respiratory tract infections. Group A streptococci release a number of soluble products which act as immunogens (e.g. streptolysin

O and streptokinase), and antibodies to these are detected in a rising titre following infection in most patients. It has been found, however, that patients with
rheumatic fever, as a group, have higher levels of such antibodies, and that their
levels remain elevated for prolonged periods compared with patients with streptococcal infections who do not develop rheumatic fever. This specific immune
hyper-reactivity is thought to result from repeated re-infection with a different
type-specific organism (rather than a result of a hyper-reactive immune status),
and it has been suggested that patients with rheumatic fever are unduly susceptible to recurrent streptococcal infections. There is some evidence that susceptibility to rheumatic fever is related to genetically determined salivary secretor
status (non-secretor being significantly more susceptible) and that blood group
O is associated with a degree of protection (Glynn *et al.*, 1959), although
the relationship of these 'markers' to protective immunity is unclear. The
observation that the incidence of rheumatic fever is reduced by the use of
anti-microbial drugs for early treatment of streptococcal respiratory infections,
and by continuous prophylaxis, further substantiates the aetiological role of
streptococci.

Rheumatic fever is characterized clinically by a febrile illness with a 'flitting'
polyarthritis, nodules, skin rashes and pancarditis. The presence of Aschoff's
nodes on tissue microscopy is widely regarded as being an important pathological
feature of the disease. These lesions consist of a perivascular granuloma of
fibrinoid material surrounded by mononuclear and multinucleated cells. The
fibrinoid material was originally thought to represent degenerating collagen, but
recent studies have emphasized the generally unidentifiable or heterogeneous
nature of fibrinoid in these and other lesions. The cells have the characteristics of mononuclear phagocytes. Aschoff's nodes have been found not only
during clinically active disease, but also in the auricular appendages of
the left atrium obtained during mitral valve surgery in patients with apparently
clinically inactive disease, emphasizing the very chronic nature of the tissue
lesions.

The evolution of tissue lesions of rheumatic fever remains incompletely
understood, although the initiating role of streptococci is undoubted. Repeated
injections of whole streptococci into the skin of rabbits (using different types of
group A streptococci) was shown by Murphy and Swift (1949) to lead to a myo-
carditis, and they demonstrated the presence of granulomatous lesions resembling
Aschoff's nodes in the heart. It has been suggested that a peptidoglycan material
of streptococcal cell walls is particularly active biologically in inducing granuloma
formation and the streptococcus has a predilection for heart muscle (for references
see Alison *et al.*, 1975). Alison and his colleagues have shown that in *in vitro*
experiments macrophages cultured with cell walls of streptococci release large
quantities of lysosomal enzymes into the medium. They have postulated that
the release of enzymes *in vivo* could account for tissue lesions; furthermore, they
may also generate chemotactic activity; for example, by direct cleavage of C5
component of complement. In this way, monocytes would be attracted to the
site of the granuloma and thus set up a chronic and enhanced inflammatory
reaction.

A more widely held view attributes the cardiac lesions in rheumatic fever to the direct cytotoxic action of anti-myocardial antibodies which are found in these patients and are believed to arise as a direct result of streptococcal infections. It has been shown that streptococci share antigens with myocardial tissue, and it is suggested that the streptococcal infection bypasses tolerance to auto-antigens in heart muscle, thereby leading to the emergence of such antibodies (Chapter 1, section on 'Cellular mechanisms of autoimmunity'). Antisera to group A streptococci raised in rabbits have been shown to cross-react with muscle tissues, confirming this view.

Anti-myocardial antibodies in the sera of patients with rheumatic fever are found to give rise to a subsarcolemmal immunofluorescent staining pattern (Hess *et al.*, 1964). Muscle-fixed IgG and complement in sections of auricular appendages in patients with rheumatic mitral valve disease obtained at the time of surgery and in the heart muscle of all chambers in fatal cases of rheumatic fever have also been documented by Kaplan and Dellenbach (1961), suggesting *in vivo* reactivity of such autoantibodies. Doubts about the pathogenicity of anti-myocardial antibodies have been expressed on the grounds that a large number of patients after myocardial infarction or cardiac surgery have serum antibodies which are apparently innocuous. However, it has been found that the antigen specificity of anti-myocardial antibodies in such patients differs from those in rheumatic fever as shown by a diffuse pattern of staining of muscle cells, as well as by their different absorption characteristics. Thus, antibodies in sera from rheumatic fever patients are absorbed by streptococci whereas those in post-cardiotomy and post-infarction sera are not; both are absorbed by myocardial extracts (Zabriskie *et al.*, 1971). In studies in which anti-myocardial antibodies in rats were produced by immunization with homologous myocardial muscle antigen, severe muscle damage was observed if an otherwise non-toxic dose of isoproterenol was administered (Gazenfeld *et al.*, 1966). In this situation, it is postulated that the myocardial cell is initially damaged non-specifically, and thus allows access to specific autoantibody to important antigenic sites where its cytotoxicity is fully expressed. It is tempting to postulate that an interplay of similar mechanisms may occur in rheumatic fever but that the non-specific injury phase is ascribable to the streptococcus as well.

Cross-reaction of anti-streptococcal antibodies with heart muscle of course does not explain other characteristic features of the disease, namely involvement of heart valves, the endocardium, the flitting arthritis and the skin rashes. It is of interest that Kingston and Glynn (1971) have been able to demonstrate that some anti-streptococcal antibodies cross-react with the endothelium and fibroblasts of the heart valve, endothelium of capillaries, synovial lining cells and the fibroblasts in the dermis as well as the myoepithelial cells of sweat glands. In addition, a reaction with astrocytes in brain tissue was shown, a finding of some relevance to the association of Sydenham's chorea with rheumatic carditis and the relationship of the condition to streptococcal infections. Whether these antibodies prove to be of pathogenetic importance for such a variety of clinico-pathological lesions remains to be proven, as does the type of allergic response which might be involved. It is difficult, for example, to explain the remarkable clinical phenomenon of erythema marginatum with its unique spreading quality. Indeed the view that these cross-reacting antibodies are merely an epiphenom-

enon has to be considered and other possible relationships between the streptococcus and disease sought.

Meningococcal arthritis

The possibility that meningococcal arthritis was a manifestation of an allergic
disorder was suspected ever since it was realized that meningococci were only
rarely isolated from joints in this condition (Pinals and Ropes, 1964). It has been
estimated that up to 10 per cent of patients suffering from meningococcal
meningitis develop an arthritis, usually involving the large joints and running a
self-limiting course. Using the technique of immunoelectrophoresis, Greenwood
and his colleagues working in Nigeria (1973) found meningococcal polysaccharide group A antigen present in the blood of 13·5 per cent of patients with
meningitis. They were struck by the high prevalence of arthritis in the anti-
genaemic group in contrast to patients with meningitis who did not show
antigenaemia. In 13 patients studied in some detail, these workers found that
arthritis usually became manifest at the stage when antigen disappeared from the
blood within 5 days or so and was followed by the appearance of antibodies. In
2 of 4 patients studied in yet further detail, levels of C3 component of complement were shown to fall significantly on the sixth day, coinciding with the
disappearance of antigen, appearance of antibody and the onset of arthritis.
This pattern of immunological abnormalities led Greenwood to postulate an
immune-complex-mediated arthritis of the type seen in acute serum sickness in
rabbits. Deposits of C3 and IgG, as well as meningococcal antigen in synovial
fluid leucocytes and in the synovial membrane, were found and thought to be
consistent with this hypothesis. Studies on skin lesions seen in these patients
also showed a vasculitis with histopathological features resembling an Arthus
reaction and, in one of the cases studied, C3, IgG and meningococcal antigen
were also demonstrable in the skin section.

In this case, the self-limiting nature of the arthritis is explained by the eventual
clearance of meningococcal antigens and disappearance of the inciting immune
complexes from the circulation. In patients developing arthritis and vasculitis,
the mechanism of inefficient antigen clearance, as well as the production of
potentially toxic immune complexes and their predilection for certain structures
in the body, remains unexplained. The disease, being self-limiting, in no way
resembles the chronic synovitis seen in rheumatoid arthritis, but nevertheless
provides an interesting model of an immunologically mediated synovitis caused
by a known infectious agent. The synovial pathology (although presumably
immune complex mediated) does not show the characteristic infiltration expected
with polymorphs, but instead shows dilated blood vessels and infiltration with
mononuclear cells.

Arthritis associated with hepatitis B infections

The identification of Australia antigen, which is believed to be the outer coat
of the hepatitis B virus and which is readily detected by immunological methods,

has provided an opportunity for understanding the pathogenesis of yet another kind of arthritis seen in association with infections. Some patients with hepatitis B virus infections develop a polyarthritis in the pre-icteric phase of the illness. In a few patients in whom the composition of the cellular exudate of the synovial fluid was studied, it was found that large mononuclear cells resembling histiocytes or macrophages were present, resembling the cells described in rubella arthritis (Chambers and Bywaters, 1963). Sera of patients who developed arthritis have been found to contain Australia antigen initially, followed by the appearance of antibody and depressed complement levels, the latter coinciding with the appearance of arthritis. Depressed complement levels were also noted in joint fluids (Onion *et al.*, 1971). Circulating immune complexes of Australia antigen with its antibody have also been documented in patients with hepatitis B infection (Almeida and Waterson, 1969). The antigen has been demonstrated in synovial membrane (Schmacher and Gall, 1974) and it is suggested that, in patients who develop an arthritis, circulating immune complexes deposit in the joint and initiate inflammation through mechanisms involving complement in a manner similar to that presumably observed in the meningococcal disease, serum sickness and systemic lupus erythematosus. The depression of complement components was found by Alpert and Schur (1971) to resemble the pattern expected from classical activation by immune complexes. The possibility that Australia antigen may itself activate complement has been excluded by investigating its effects on complement *in vitro*.

References

AHO, K., AHVONEN, P., ALKIO, P., LASSUS, A., SAIRANEN, E., SIEVERS, K. and TIILIKAINEN, A. (1975). *Ann. rheum. Dis.* (Suppl.), **34**, 29.

ALISON, A. C., CARDELLA, C. and DAVIES, P. (1975). *Rheumatology*, **6**, 251.

ALMEIDA, J. and WATERSON, A. P. (1969). *Lancet*, **2**, 983.

ALPERT, E. and SCHUR, P. H. (1971). *New Engl. J. Med.*, **285**, 185.

BACON, P. A., BLUESTONE, R., GOLDBERG, L. S., WEBB, F. W., PEARSON, C. M., COOKE, M. and STEVENS, J. G. (1974). *Ann. rheum. Dis.*, **33**, 413.

CHAMBERS, R. J. and BYWATERS, E. G. L. (1963). *Ann. rheum. Dis.*, **22**, 263.

DECKER, J. L. and BARDEN, J. A. (1975). *Rheumatology*, **6**, 338.

GAZENFIELD, E., ROSENMANN, E., DAVIES, A. M. and LAUFER, A. (1966). *Immunology*, **10**, 193.

GLYNN, L. E. (1975). In *Clinical Aspects of Immunology*, 3rd edn., p. 1079. Ed. P. G. H. Gell, R. R. A. Coombs and P. J. Lachmann. Blackwell Scientific Publications, Oxford.

GLYNN, A. A., GLYNN, L. E. and HOLBOROW, E. J. (1959). *Brit. med. J.* **2**, 266.

GREENWOOD, B. M., WHITTLE, H. C. and BRYCESON, A. D. M. (1973). *Brit. med. J.*, **2**, 737.

HESS, E. V., FINK, C. W., TARANTA, A. and ZIFF, M. (1964). *J. clin. Invest.*, **43**, 886.

KAPLAN, M. H. and DALLENBACH, F. D. (1961). *J. exp. Med.*, **113**, 1.

KINGSTON, D. and GLYNN, L. E. (1971). *Immunology*, **21**, 1003.

MURPHY, G. E. and SWIFT, H. F. (1949). *J. exp. Med.*, **89**, 687.

ONION, D. K., CRUMPACKER, C. S. and GILLILAND, B. D. (1971). *Ann. intern. Med.*, **75**, 29.

PINALS, R. A. and ROPES, W. W. (1964). *Arthr. and Rheum.*, 7, 241.
SCHUMACHER, H. R. and GALL, E. P. (1974). *Amer. J. Med.*, 57, 655.
SMITH, J. W. and SANFORD, J. P. (1967). *Ann. intern. Med.*, **67**, 651.
ZABRISKIE, J. B., READ, S. E. and ELLIS, R. J. (1971). In *Progress in Immunology*, Vol. 1, p. 216. Ed. B. Amos. Academic Press, New York and London.

11

Vasculitis and Polyarteritis Nodosa

Vasculitis: definition; classification; pathogenesis

The term 'vasculitis' describes an ill-defined clinicopathological entity and is sometimes used as a generic term for all types of conditions in which the vessel walls show evidence of vascular damage initiated by an inflammatory process. Any type and size of vessel may be involved, and signs of damage and inflammation are assessed by clinical criteria and evidence of structural alteration in blood vessels (see Chapter 2). The histopathological signs of active inflammation in vasculitis depend, to a certain extent, on the type of vessel involved; for example, when it involves capillaries it is evidenced by dilatation and cellular emigration (described as 'perivascular infiltration'), whereas in larger vessels there may be evidence of polymorph or mononuclear cell infiltration of the wall as well as evidence of fibrinoid necrosis and damage to collagen. Evidence of changes compatible with previous inflammatory reaction may also be acceptable, but are less specific and often impossible to distinguish from degenerative change; for example fibrosis of the media of arteries, unless accompanied by interruption of disappearance of the internal elastic lamina. The basis of pathogenesis of certain other vascular lesions is also poorly understood but could have resulted from inflammation; for example, intimal hyperplasia and intravascular thrombosis. The use of immunofluorescent stains for immunoglobulin and complement, as well as ultrastructural examination, sometimes shows evidence of immune deposits which are not evident on light microscopy, and provide a better basis for understanding of the pathophysiology of certain diseases.

In practice, a diagnosis of vasculitis is often made on the basis of well recognized clinical syndromes with the aid of microscopy of tissues, when practical. Although, strictly speaking, inflammation of synovium in rheumatoid arthritis is due to a vasculitis as is the widespread and diverse multi-system disease of systemic lupus erythematosus, in this chapter only certain specific types of diseases of vessels occurring with rheumatic disease, or as primary abnormalities, are included as examples for the purposes of discussing immune pathogenesis.

In the majority of patients no initiating agent is discovered, although typical lesions of vasculitis have occurred in conjunction with infections (for example, meningococcal septicaemia, erythema nodosum leprosum, secondary syphilis and virus hepatitis) and exposure to drugs and administration of serum proteins. In these conditions evidence for circulating immune complexes with participation of complement activation has been obtained (see Chapters 2 and 10). It is of interest that some of these patients also develop a polyarthritis, although in general the reason why certain organs are involved, whilst others are spared, remains problematical. These diseases allow a study of the composition of the complexes and the nature of defects of immune regulation which result in an inefficient clearance of antigen. In the vasculitis seen in erythema nodosum leprosum, for example, the marked depression of specific (and less marked non-specific) cellular immunity is accompanied by an exaggerated humoral response to the mycobacteria and emergence of autoimmunity (Turk, 1970). The type of cellular defects which may be of importance are discussed in Chapter 1; they show some parallel with certain rheumatic diseases also characterized by depression of cellular immunity and stimulation of autoimmunity and formation of immune complexes.

Attempts have been made to classify vasculitis on the basis of vessel size involved—i.e. large, middle or small arteries, arterioles, capillaries and venules. Some syndromes do characteristically involve certain sized blood vessels; thus polyarteritis nodosa is a disease of medium-sized or small arteries and Henoch–Schönlein purpura affects capillaries and venules (see Table 11.1). Such a classification may be too restrictive, however, since different sized vessels are sometimes involved even in these diseases (e.g. glomerulitis in polyarteritis nodosa), and is in any case not specific enough, since the same type of vessel disease may be seen in more than one syndrome (e.g. lesions resembling polyarteritis occur in patients with rheumatoid arthritis).

The fact that immune complexes mediate vascular damage is regarded as a possible unifying concept of pathogenesis for all forms of vasculitis. The advances in methodology of detection of complexes and complement components in the circulation, and when fixed to tissues, (Chapter 4) have contributed much to these ideas. However, such abnormalities cannot always be detected, although it is realized that, soon after tissue fixation, complexes and complement tend to be removed by phagocytosis or obscured by the inflammatory reaction (Cream *et al.*, 1971; Cochrane and Koffler, 1973). The possibility that hitherto unexplored cellular immune reactions may be of direct importance in mediating certain forms of vasculitis has been raised by the finding of cell-mediated immunity to muscle and arterial wall antigens in temporal arteritis (Esiri *et al.*, 1973; Hazelman *et al.*, 1975).

Vasculitis in rheumatoid arthritis

In rheumatoid arthritis attention has been drawn to at least two different types of vascular disease, both of which tend to occur in patients with long-standing disease with nodules and a high titre of rheumatoid factor:

1. affecting the digital blood vessels, characterized pathologically by intimal hyperplasia (Scott *et al.*, 1961) without any evidence of inflammatory reaction or demonstration of immune complexes or complement in the vessel wall;

Table 11.1   Inflammatory vascular disease

Syndrome	Distribution of lesions	Size of vessel	Histology	Evidence of autoimmunity or immune complexes in vessels
Vasculitis complicating rheumatoid arthritis and other connective tissue disease	Digital vessels, peripheral nerves, myocardial, pericardial, mesenteric and kidney vessels	Medium to small arteries	Fibrinoid necrosis with polymorph and mononuclear cell infiltrates	Hypocomplementaemia. Cryoglobulinaemia. Immunoglobulin and complement detected in vessel walls. Autoantibodies usually present
Polyarteritis nodosa	Kidney, heart, liver, gastrointestinal tract, pancreas, striated muscle, peripheral nerves, testis, skin, lungs	Medium to small arteries	Fibrinoid necrosis beginning in the media, neutrophil and eosinophil infiltrates, with subsequent lymphocyte and plasma cell infiltration and fibroblast proliferation. Lesions focal	Immunoglobulin and complement detected, in some lesions with Australia antigen. Autoantibodies not a feature
Giant cell arteritis	Cranial, mesenteric, coronary and limb vessels	Medium to small arteries	Intima involved usually with lymphocyte, macrophage and giant cells	Immunoglobulin and complement have not been found associated with temporal artery lesions. Cellular immunity to muscle, vascular antigens
Takayashu's disease	Aortic arch and its branches		Adventitial inflammatory response with mononuclear and giant cell infiltrates	Occasionally positive anti-nuclear factors, anti-aortic antibodies reported
Wegener's granulomatosis	Nasal and palatal tissues, lungs, kidneys, spleen and skin	Medium to small arteries	As for Takayashu's disease; but, in addition to distribution, distinguished by greater vessel necrosis and granuloma formation. Giant cells and eosinophils may be seen	Immunoglobulin and electron-dense deposits detectable in involved kidneys
Behcet's syndrome	Skin, joint, mucous membranes, CNS	Large, medium and small vessels	Arterial lesions with acute and chronic inflammatory cells	
Henoch–Schönlein purpura	Skin, joint, bowel, kidneys	Capillaries and venules	Cutaneous vasculitis and focal glomerulonephritis	Immunoglobulin and complement in cutaneous vessels. 'Granular' Ig on immunofluorescence and electron-dense kidney deposits on electron microscopy. Autoantibodies and hypocomplementaemia rare

2. the occurrence of a lesion similar to polyarteritis nodosa, consisting of necrotizing arteritis and involving the blood vessels to viscera, sclera and nerves and presenting as infarction of the affected organs, scleritis or neuropathy, respectively.

The two types of lesion can co-exist in the same patient. However, the former lesion is commoner and clinically often relatively benign. In patients with the latter type of lesion cryoglobulinaemia has been documented by Weisman and Zvaifler (1975) in many instances. Relative hypocomplementaemia also occurs and may sometimes be obvious and show the classical pattern of depletion of serum complement components C1, C4 and C3. In one study this hypocomplementaemic pattern was found in 9 of 13 patients with cutaneous vasculitis occurring as a complication of SLE, RA or Sjögren's syndrome (Soter *et al.*, 1974). Complement proteins and immunoglobulin have been found in the vasa nervosum in rheumatoid arthritis (Conn *et al.*, 1972). The relevance of the occurrence of rheumatoid factors in vasculitis is discussed in Chapter 5, 'Rheumatoid Arthritis'. The finding of immune complexes by reaction with radio-labelled C1q by Lambert and his colleagues (1975) raises the possibility that circulating immune complexes are not an uncommon occurrence in rheumatoid arthritis (see Chapter 5); their precise relationship to the causation of vascular damage is therefore not clearly understood and requires further study.

The occurrence of purpura in some patients with rheumatoid arthritis coincides with the presence of intermediate-sized complexes (9–17S) in the sera of the type seen without arthritis (Capra *et al.*, 1971). These purpuric lesions have been regarded to be of a vasculitic nature by some authors. This type of lesion thus provides a third form of vascular complication occurring in rheumatoid arthritis.

Vasculitis in other connective tissue diseases

In systemic lupus erythematosus the immune complex mediation of the multi-system disease is widely established and raises a semantic problem since it may be said that the manifestations of the disease are all due to a vasculitis. Occasional patients are, however, found at autopsy to have widespread necrotizing arteritis (Karani, 1953; Muehrcke *et al.*, 1957). Digital occlusive disease of the Raynaud's phenomenon type as well as that due to organic occlusion occurs, and probably resembles the disease seen in rheumatoid arthritis.

In scleroderma and dermatomyositis, Raynaud's phenomenon is almost invariable. This may be based partially on vasospasm but is also accompanied by occlusive disease. The nature of the occlusive disease, however, is uncertain since, by the time the vessels are examined, disease has been present for a long time and changes may have occurred as a result of thrombosis and revascularization. Calcinosis in blood vessel walls and soft-tissue ectopic calcification occur in such patients. A well documented arteritis involving the medium-sized renal and pulmonary vessels has been described in patients with scleroderma. In dermatomyositis, especially in childhood, the blood vessels in the muscles show evidence of immune complex deposition (Chapter 8).

Polyarteritis nodosa

Polyarteritis nodosa is a disorder of unknown cause characterized by inflammation and necrosis in the walls of medium-sized or small arteries. It was first described just over a hundred years ago by Kusmow and Mayer who used the term 'periarteritis nodosa' to describe a type of case with intimal inflammation in medium-sized arteries leading to nodular aneurysms which could be palpated under the skin of the trunk or extremities, with similar lesions observed at autopsy in organs. Rose and Spencer (1957) analysed 111 cases of polyarteritis nodosa. They were able to divide most of their cases into two groups: (1) with, and (2) without lung involvement. Those with lung involvement (which were about one-third of the number studied) suffered from an illness characterized by bronchitis, asthma or pneumonia, often preceding a more generalized systemic disease. Such patients frequently showed eosinophilia, and midline granulomas of the upper respiratory tract were observed in some. The lung lesions at autopsy consisted of large necrotic and caseous lesions, atypical consolidations, infarcts or bronchiectasis. Evidence of polyarteritis with the typical eosinophil and giant cell infiltration were observed not only in lung vessels but also in other parts of the body. Hypertension and renal involvement were more common in the second group of patients. Polyarteritis nodosa is not usually accompanied by an observable polyarthritis although pains in muscles are not uncommon.

It has already been pointed out that histologically indistinguishable lesions occur in some patients with rheumatoid arthritis and other connective tissue diseases. It is possible that the common denominator for all these lesions is the presence of a special type of circulating immune complex. Circulating immune complexes have been implicated in the pathogenesis of arteritis in experimental serum sickness, and in the Aleutian mink an immune-complex-mediated arteritis is accompanied by para-proteinaemia and lymphoma. In polyarteritis nodosa, up to 30 per cent of patients were found to possess circulating immune complexes which contained Australia antigen (Gocke *et al.*, 1970). A similar association was found by other workers, but has not been consistently confirmed (Prince and Trepo, 1971). Australia antigen–antibody complexes in these patients are presumably different from those observed in patients in the prodromal phase of Australia-antigen-positive hepatitis who developed polyarthritis (Chapter 8). However, a link with polyarteritis nodosa exists since some patients with Australia-antigen-positive hepatitis develop necrotizing arteritis.

The role of arterial hypertension in the pathogenesis of polyarteritis has been suggested by the finding of fibrinoid necrosis in the vessel walls of patients suffering from malignant hypertension. Necrotizing arteritis also followed a rapidly rising blood pressure in the rat (Smith and Zeek, 1947) and in the rabbit (Campbell and Santos-Butch, 1959). However, the lesions in human polyarteritis do not have to be accompanied by hypertension. Pressure changes may nevertheless be of importance in the deposition of immune complexes in vessel walls (see Chapter 2).

Giant cell (temporal) arteritis

Giant cell arteritis is characterized by a granulomatous inflammation of large arteries, the vessels of the internal and external carotid systems frequently being involved. The classical onset is with pain in the head and face, and symptoms of cerebral ischaemia may be pronounced. A polymyalgia rheumatica type of syndrome is usual and may be the sole manifestation of giant cell arteritis. In this condition immune complexes or complement deposits have not been demonstrated in the vessel walls. A recent report has suggested the possibility that cellular reactions to muscle homogenates and vascular antigens may be of importance (Hazelman *et al.*, 1975).

Pulseless disease

Takayashu described a syndrome affecting young women, in which the aortic arch is involved by an inflammatory giant cell arteritis. Patients may also show systemic involvement (Strachan, 1964). Although histologically similar to giant cell arteritis, its exclusive occurrence in women of a young age group contrasts with the elderly patients with the former condition. Moreover, in patients with Takayashu's disease autoantibodies are often present in blood.

Wegener's granulomatosis

Wegener's granulomatosis is a rare disorder characterized by the presence of ulcerating lesions of the respiratory tract which may be accompanied by a widespread vasculitis and glomerulonephritis. The lesions in the respiratory tract may be initially confined to the upper tract, and, in this situation, tend to occur in the 'midline' of the palate or in the nasal septum (hence termed 'midline granuloma') or involve the sinuses. Such lesions may be associated with or followed by severe destructive lesions in the lung. The respiratory disease may also be complicated by a systemic vasculitis and glomerulonephritis.

Clinically, the patients may present with a variety of respiratory symptoms and signs, as well as skin lesions, fever, arthralgias, renal failure and systemic vascular occlusive disease. The respiratory 'granuloma' shows changes of an inflammatory exudate in which mononuclear cells, plasma cells, eosinophils and giant cells may be seen and is accompanied by a 'vasculitis' characterized by vessel wall necrosis with a predominantly polymorphonuclear cellular infiltration (Walton, 1958; Carrington and Liebow, 1966). The relationship of lung involvement in Wegener's granulomatosis to polyarteritis lesions of lung, and of the upper respiratory tract granuloma to malignant granuloma of the nose, is not clear, and, in some instances at least, are the one and the same disorder. Renal changes are those of a focal and segmental glomerulonephritis with necrosis. Medium-sized and smaller arteries and veins of other organs may be involved in a generalized vascular disease, the lesions resembling polyarteritis nodosa but showing a tendency towards simultaneous arterial and venous involvement.

The aetiology of Wegener's granulomatosis is unknown but the appearance of the disseminated vascular lesions (when these occur) suggests a 'serum sickness' type of circulating immune complex disease. The finding of IgG and C3 with a coarse granular pattern along the glomerular basement membrane in some renal biopsies supports this view, but serum complement levels are normal or raised (Fauci and Wolff, 1973). In 2 of 10 patients studied by electron microscopy in one study, electron-dense deposits resembling immune complexes were detected in the subepithelial position, whilst in the rest sclerosis of segments of glomeruli or no change were recorded (Horn *et al.*, 1974).

A notable therapeutic response to cyclophosphamide (Fauci *et al.*, 1971) distinguishes Wegener's granulomatosis from other forms of vasculitis in which the effect of cytostatic drugs is less predictable.

Behcet's syndrome

The clinical and histological features of Behcet's syndrome are also largely due to an underlying vasculitis (see Table 11.1).

Henoch–Schönlein purpura

Henoch–Schönlein purpura, a disease principally of childhood, is characterized clinically by purpura, arthritis and abdominal pain. Renal disease is present in up to half of the patients (see Table 11.1). Serum complement levels (β_{1C} and CH_{50}) and anti-nuclear antibodies have not been found to be abnormal although studies have been less extensive than in the adult counterpart (Cream *et al.*, 1970; Gary *et al.*, 1972). Homozygous C2 deficiency has been described in one individual with Henoch–Schönlein purpura, in whom mycoplasmas were demonstrated in serum (Sussman *et al.*, 1973).

Studies of kidney biopsies have been reported to show granular or nodular deposits of immunoglobulin and complement (β_{1C}), particularly in the mesangium and to a lesser extent in the glomerular basement membrane (Urzar *et al.*, 1968). Although the disease reportedly follows infections, specific organisms have not been well defined.

References

CAMPBELL, W. G. and SANTOS-BUCH, C. A. (1959). *Amer. J. Path.*, **35**, 769.

CAPRA, J. D., WINCHESTER, R. J. and KUNKEL, H. G. (1971). *Medicine (Baltimore)*, **50**, 128.

CARRINGTON, C. B. and LIEBOW, A. A. (1966). *Amer. J. Med.*, **41**, 497.

COCHRANE, C. G. and KOFFLER, D. (1973). *Adv. Immunol.*, **16**, 185.

CONN, D. L., MCDUFFIE, F. C. and DYCK, P. J. (1972). *Arthr. and Rheum.* **15**, 135.

CREAM, J. J. GUMPEL, J. M. and PEACHEY, R. D. G. (1970). *Quart. J. Med. (N.S.)*, **39**, 461.

CREAM, J. J., BRYCESON, A. D. M. and RYDER, G. (1971). *Brit. J. Derm.*, **84**, 106.

ESIRI, M. M., MACLENNAN, I. M. and HAZELMAN, B. L. (1973). *Clin. exp. Immunol.*, **14**, 25.

FAUCI, A. S., WOLFF, S. and JOHNSON, J. S. (1971). *New Engl. J. Med.*, **285**, 1493.

FAUCI, A. S. and WOLFF, S. M. (1973). *Medicine (Baltimore)*, **52**, 535.

GARY, N. E., MAZZARA, J. T. and HOLFOLDER, L. (1972). *Ann. intern. Med.*, **229**, 234.

GOCKE, D. J., HSU, K., MORGAN, G., BOMBARDIERI, S., LOCKSHIN, M. and CHRISTIAN, C. L. (1970), *Lancet*, **2**, 1149.

HAZELMAN, B. L., MCLENNAN, I. C. M. and ESIRI, M. M. (1975). *Ann. rheum. Dis.*, **34**, 122.

HORN, R. G., FAUCI, A. S., ROSENTHAL, A. S. and WOLFF, S. M. (1974). *Am. J. Path.*, **74**, 423.

KARANI, S. (1953). *Postgrad. med. J.*, **29**, 321.

LAMBERT, P. H., NYEDEGGER, U. E., PERRIN, L. H., MCCORMICK, J., FEHR, K. and MIESCHER, P. A. (1975). In *Rheumatology*, Vol. 6, p. 52. Ed. S. Karger, Basel.

MUEHRCKE, R. C., KARK, R. M. M., PIRANI, C. L. and POLLAK, V. E. (1975). *Medicine (Baltimore)*, **36**, 145.

PRINCE, A. M. and TREPO, C. (1971). *Lancet*, **1**, 1309.

ROSE, G. A. and SPENCER, H. (1957). *Quart. J. Med. (N.S.)*, **26**, 43.

SCOTT, J. T., HOURIHANE, D. O., DOYLE, F. H., STEINER, R. E., LAWS, J. W., DIXON, A. and BYWATERS, E. G. L. (1961). *Ann. rheum. Dis.*, **20**, 224.

SMITH, C. C. and ZEEK, P. M. (1947). *Amer. J. Path.*, **23**, 147.

SOTER, N. A., AUSTEN, K. F. and GIGLI, E. (1974). *J. invest. Derm.*, **63**, 219.

STRACHAN, R. W. (1964). *Quart. J. Med. (N.S.)*, **33**, 57.

SUSSMAN, M., JONES, J. H., ALMEIDA, J. D. and LACHMANN, P. J. (1973). *Clin. exp. Immunol.*, **14**, 531.

TURK, J. L. (1970). In *Immune Complex Diseases*, p. 165. Ed. L. Bonomo and J. L. Turk. Carlo Erba Foundation, Milan.

URIZAR, R. E., MICHAEL, A., SISSON, S. and VERNIER, R. L. (1968). *Lab. Invest.*, **19**, 437.

WALTON, E. W. (1958). *Brit. med. J.*, **2**, 265.

WEISMAN, M. and ZVAIFLER, N. (1975). *J. clin. Invest.*, **56**, 725.

12

Therapeutic Implications

Immunosuppression

The role of humoral and cell-mediated immune responses in the production of inflammation and tissue damage has been established or strongly suspected in a number of diseases discussed in this book. These pathogenetic concepts have prompted the belief that manipulations resulting in a suppression of an established immune response may prove to be of therapeutic benefit. Ideally, immuno-suppression should be specific for the component suspected to be involved in pathogenesis, but in practice is non-specific since it is usually achieved by removal of antibody and immunologically committed cells, or by a reduction in the numbers (or metabolic activity) of cells involved in antibody synthesis and mediating cellular immunity. Whilst removal of antigen–antibody complexes (e.g. by plasmapheresis) and of lymphocytes (e.g. by thoracic duct drainage) represent interesting examples of a logical means of achieving immunosuppression, these manoeuvres do not correct the immunological abnormality and are still largely experimental, although therapeutic successes have been claimed, for example, following thoracic duct drainage of lymphocytes in patients with rheumatoid arthritis (Paulus *et al.*, 1973). On the other hand, a number of drugs believed to possess immunosuppressive activity have been used extensively in the treatment of rheumatic diseases, including corticosteroids, alkylating agents (e.g. cyclophosphamide and chlorambucil), purine analogues (e.g. azathioprine) and folic acid antagonists (e.g. methotrexate).

There is a considerable amount of evidence that the above-mentioned drugs achieve an operationally defined state of immunosuppression, for example, leading to prolongation of allograft survival, diminution of protective immunity against infections, and depression of antibody- and cell-mediated responses (at least in experimental animals). Their mode of action is, however, complex and poorly understood. For example, it involves action at multiple sites of the on-going immune response, as well as influencing mediators of inflammation. Thus corticosteroids are powerful anti-inflammatory agents, influence T and B cell function and their circulation, but also lower the numbers of blood monocytes (reviewed by Berenbaum, 1975). Cyclophosphamide, in high doses, selectively depletes B cells in lymphoid tissues but, if given before antigen, inhibits both antibody synthesis and delayed hypersensitivity; paradoxically, it may enhance contact sensitivity due to loss of B cell regulatory mechanisms (Turk *et al.*, 1972). In the rat, immunosuppressive agents are also anti-inflammatory (Currey, 1971). It might be further anticipated that cytostatic drugs could influence the course of those rheumatic diseases for which a viral aetiology is suspected by virtue of their action on virus nucleic acid metabolism (an 'anti-viral' effect). In practice, in patients receiving cytostatic drugs, immune responses have been found to be depressed (Winkelstein *et al.*, 1972) or unaltered (Denman *et al.*, 1970; Curtis *et al.*, 1973), thus further questioning the validity of the idea that the drugs are merely immunosuppressive in their action.

Cytostatic drugs in connective tissue diseases

RHEUMATOID ARTHRITIS

The use of cytostatic drugs in rheumatoid arthritis has, in general, proven to be of benefit (reviewed by Currey, 1975). Azathioprine or cyclophosphamide, started relatively early in the course of rheumatoid arthritis, were equally effective and similar in their efficacy to gold therapy (see Currey, 1975). A controlled trial of cyclophosphamide conducted by co-operating centres under the auspices of the American Rheumatism Association (1970) showed it to be of benefit. In both these trials, the rate of progression of joint damage assessed radiologically was slowed. In cases with severe rheumatoid arthritis receiving corticosteroids, the use of azathioprine led to a 36 per cent lowering of the steroid dosage (Mason *et al.*, 1969). Although immunosuppressive agents might be expected to be particularly beneficial in rheumatoid patients with vasculitis, a preliminary controlled trial with azathioprine did not demonstrate such benefit, mainly because of the spontaneously fluctuating course of vasculitis and a relatively good prognosis of the control group (Nicholls *et al.*, 1973). The drop in levels of cryoglobulin and apparent improvement in patients with rheumatoid vasculitis following cyclophosphamide have, however, been documented (Weismann and Zvaifler, 1975) and suggest that further trials are necessary.

SYSTEMIC LUPUS ERYTHEMATOSUS

The results of the use of cytostatic drugs in SLE are controversial for several reasons. For example, it is recognized that the outlook of patients is not entirely determined by their immunological disorder but has been considerably improved by the availability of effective antibiotics, diuretics, anti-hypertensive drugs and the use of steroids (their anti-inflammatory effect being perhaps most relevant). Any fair trial of cytostatic drugs requires that the group receiving treatment should be as similar as possible to the control group. This creates great difficulties since the clinical patterns of multi-system disease in SLE are extremely heterogeneous, and it almost certainly includes patients whose natural prognosis is also extremely variable. Such a problem is self-evident even in SLE patients with active renal disease since it has been shown that the prognosis of patients with a diffuse glomerulonephritis is worse than that of patients with focal or membranous nephropathy (Chapter 7).

There is a very large number of uncontrolled reports of the apparently beneficial effects of immunosuppressive agents in SLE. In many of the reported studies, immunological abnormalities were usually completely corrected. The situation is, however, confused by a lack of impressive data in controlled trials. Cyclophosphamide, together with steroids, has been shown in a short-term trial to be better than steroids alone or azathioprine and steroids in treatment with lupus nephritis, although it appeared to have little beneficial effect in patients with severe impairment of glomerular function (Steinberg *et al.*, 1971; Steinberg and Decker, 1974). In 38 patients grouped similarly in a randomized study from the same centre, followed for a mean of $2\frac{1}{2}$ years, gradual deterioration in renal function was observed in all three groups (i.e. cyclophosphamide plus steroids, steroids alone, and azathioprine plus steroids) but was most marked in patients treated with steroids only (Decker *et al.*, 1975). Of 12 patients treated with cyclophosphamide, no patient died as a result of SLE or required dialysis for renal failure (1 died of infection and 1 of pulmonary embolus), whereas amongst patients treated only with steroids 3 died of lupus nephritis, 2 required dialysis, and 3 died of CNS complications. Azathioprine-treated patients included 2 with progressive renal disease resulting in death (1 patient) or long-term dialysis (1 patient). Infections, sometimes fatal, occurred in patients on cytotoxic drugs. The authors concluded that although cyclophosphamide appeared to be superior to azathioprine (added to steroids), both were of marginal value compared to steroids alone, and that other forms of treatment schedules should be investigated. In a study of 22 patients (Garancis and Piering, 1973) with biopsy-proven glomerulonephritis, no deaths occurred in the cyclophosphamide-treated group compared with 4 deaths in the group treated with azathioprine (prednisolone given in doses less than 10 mg daily to both groups).

Sztejnbok *et al.* (1973) found that, of 16 patients treated over a period of 3 years with azathioprine and any necessary amount of steroids, none died; this compared with 6 deaths in the group of 19 treated with only steroids. There was also evidence that in the azathioprine-treated group, hospital admissions were less frequent and the steroid dose lower than in the control group. However, the study excluded 7 patients (5 of whom had received azathioprine) who died during the first hospital admission, which may have biased the study in favour of the azathioprine-treated group. In a study comparing high-dose steroids (60–100 mg daily) or azathioprine alone, azathioprine and steroids combined and a fourth treatment group of azathioprine and heparin, patients with proliferative glomerulonephritis due to SLE did best when treated with combined treatment or azathioprine alone (Cade *et al.*, 1973). However, the mortality of the steroid-treated group was exceptionally high. In a controlled study of 16 patients with lupus nephritis treated with steroids alone, or with steroids and azathioprine, no significant difference was noted, improvement occurring in both (Donadio *et al.*, 1972). Similar results were obtained in a study lasting a longer period of 18–24 months (Hahn *et al.*, 1975).

Although it is difficult to generalize on the basis of these studies, it seems that cytostatic drug therapy may be of limited value, but may help patients with active SLE who do not respond to treatment with steroids or who require unduly high doses to maintain them free of symptoms. Although cyclophosphamide appears to be more effective than azathioprine (as it is in controlling the lupus syndrome of NZ mice; Russell *et al.*, 1966), it is also more toxic and hazardous than azathioprine (see below).

Certain authors have drawn attention to a phenomenon of rebound of disease activity following sudden cessation of cytostatic therapy and this has led to the recommendation that the drugs be withdrawn gradually or maintained as long-term therapy (Sharon *et al.*, 1973).

OTHER DISEASES

Corticosteroid-resistant dermatomyositis and polymyositis have apparently responded to treatment with methotrexate (Malaviya *et al.*, 1968; Sokoloff *et al.*, 1971). MacKenzie (1970) has reported that prolonged therapy with chlorambucil is beneficial in scleroderma.

Striking improvement in Wegener's granulomatosis, including patients with renal involvement, has been reported to occur following cyclophosphamide therapy (Fauci *et al.*, 1971).

Complications of cytostatic drug therapy

Alkylating agents, anti-metabolites and purine analogues can all give rise to serious bone marrow depression, and occasionally patients have died as a result of such complications. Patients treated with these drugs are also liable to serious infections, although the relative contributions to the patient's increased susceptibility to infections due to the disease itself and frequent concomitant steroid therapy remains difficult to evaluate. Infections with organisms such as cytomegalic virus, herpes simplex, *Mycobacterium tuberculosis* and fungi remain a distinct possibility in such patients.

The use of cyclophosphamide is accompanied by alopecia, haemorrhagic cystitis and bladder fibrosis; it may also lead to ovarian failure and azoospermia. Azathioprine is apparently free of such side effects; however, chromosomal damage has been reported with its use. Cytostatic drugs are potentially teratogenic in man, although several women on azathioprine have conceived and delivered healthy babies; its use in women of child-bearing age should be carefully considered. Methotrexate, if given repeatedly, can lead to hepatic fibrosis.

There is a 30- to 40-fold increased risk of developing lymphoma in patients receiving azathioprine and a 300-fold increased risk of developing reticulum cell sarcoma compared with the rest of the population (Hoover and Fraumeni, 1973). However, this complication appears to be especially prevalent in patients who have received kidney allografts, since very few patients receiving azathioprine for other conditions have been reported to have developed tumours, and some of these had also received alkylating agents (Weinberg, 1975). Reports of tumours in cyclophosphamide-treated patients appear to continue.

In summary, whilst cyclophosphamide appears to be clinically and immuno-logically more effective, it is also more toxic than azathioprine. It therefore seems prudent at this stage of knowledge to regard these drugs with circumspection but to be prepared to use them for potentially life-threatening complications such as progressive renal damage in SLE. It is doubtful whether they have any place in the routine management of rheumatoid arthritis, especially in view of the equivalent efficacy of the somewhat less toxic drugs, gold and D-penicillamine.

Immunostimulation of immunorestoration

The theory that autoimmunity results from defects of immunoregulation characterized by depressed cellular immunity and exaggerated humoral immunity (Chapter 1) has led to the consideration of the possibility that the cellular immune defect could be corrected therapeutically. A controlled cross-over type of trial was used to test whether rheumatoid arthritis might respond to leucocyte dialysates prepared from healthy blood containing transfer factor (Maini *et al.*, 1975), a mediator which confers specific cellular immunity of the donor to the recipient. Such treatment might also prove to be of value if patients with rheumatoid arthritis lacked specific immunity to a common virus which was present in normal individuals (e.g. rubella; see Chapter 5). In the event, improvement occurred in the early part of the trial in all patients, irrespective of whether transfer factor or saline (control) injections were administered, indicating a strong placebo effect and obscuring possible effects of transfer factor.

The drug levamisole has recently been tried in the treatment of rheumatoid arthritis on the basis that it stimulates cellular immunity in experimental situations. Preliminary results from different centres are not in agreement so far, benefit being claimed as well as negative results.

References

AMERICAN RHEUMATISM ASSOCIATION, COOPERATING CLINICS COMMITTEE OF THE (1970). *New Engl. J. Med.*, **283**, 883.

BERENBAUM, M. C. (1975). In *Progress in Immunology*, Vol. II, 5, p. 233. Ed. L. Brent and J. Holborow. North Holland Publishing Co., Amsterdam

CADE, R., SPOONER, G., SCHLEIN, E., PICKERING, M., DEQUESADA, A., HOLCOMB, A., JUNCOS, L., RICHARD, G., SHIRES, D., LEVIN, D., HACKETT, R., FREE, J., HUNT, R. and FREGLY, M. (1973), *Nephron*, **10**, 37.

CURREY, H. L. F. (1971). *Clin. exp. Immunol.*, **9**, 879.

CURREY, H. L. F. (1975). In *Progress in Immunology*, Vol. II, 5, p. 263. Ed. L. Brent and J. Holborow. North Holland Publishing Co., Amsterdam.

CURTIS, J. E., SHARP, J. T., LIDSKY, M. D. and HERSCH, E. M. (1973). *Arthr. and Rheum.* **16**, 34.

DECKER, J. L., KLIPPEL, J. H., PLOTZ, P. H. and STEINBERG, A. D. (1975). *Ann. intern. Med.*, **83**, 606.

DENMAN, E. J., DENMAN, A. M., GREENWOOD, B. M., GALL, D. and HEATH, R. B. (1970). *Ann. rheum. Dis.*, **29**, 220.

DONADIO, J. V., HOLLEY, K. E., WAGONER, R. D., FERGUSON, R. H. and McDUFFIE, F. C. (1972). *Ann. intern. Med.*, 77, 829.

FAUCI, A. S., WOLFF, S. M. and JOHNSON, J. S. (1971). *New Engl. J. Med.*, **285**, 1433.

GARANCIS, J. C. and PIERING, W. F. (1973). *Clin. Pharmacol. Ther.*, **14**, 130 (abstr.).

HAHN, B. H., KANTOR, O. S. and OSTERLAND, C. K. (1975). *Ann. intern. Med.*. **83** 597.

HOOVER, R. and FRAUMENI, J. R., Jr. (1973). *Lancet*, **2**, 55.

MACKENZIE, A. H. (1970). *Arthr. and Rheum.*, **13**, 334.

MAINI, R. N., SCOTT, J. T., ROFFE, L., HAMBLIN, A. and DUMONDE, D. C. (1975). In *Infection and Immunity*, p. 579. Ed. D. C. Dumonde. Blackwell Scientific Publications, Oxford.

MALAVIYA, A. N., MANY, A. and SCHWARTZ, R. S. (1968). *Lancet*, **2**, 485.

MASON, R. M., CURREY, H. L. F., BARNES, C. G., DUNNE, J. F., HAZELMAN, B. L. and STRICKLAND, I. D. (1969). *Brit. Med. J.*, **1**, 420.

NICHOLLS, A., SNAITH, M. L., MAINI, R. N. and SCOTT, J. T. (1973). *Ann. rheum. Dis.*, **32**, 589 (abstr.).

PAULUS, H. E., MACHLEDER, H., BANGERT, R., STRATTON, J. A., PETER, J. B., GOLDBERG, L., WHITEHOUSE, M. W., YU, D. and PEARSON, C. M. (1973). *Clin. Immunol. Immunopath.*, **1**, 173.

RUSSELL, P. J., HICKS, J. D. and BURNETT, F. M. (1966). *Lancet*, **1**, 1279.

SHARON, E., KAPLAN, D. and DIAMOND, H. S. (1973). *New Engl. J. Med.*, **288**, 122.

SOKOLOFF, M. C., GOLDBERG, L. S. and PEARSON, C. M. (1971). *Lancet*, **1**, 14.

STEINBERG, A. D. and DECKER, J. L. (1974). *Arthr. and Rheum.*, **17**, 923.

STEINBERG, A. D., KALTREIDER, B., STAPLES, P. J., GOETZL, E. J., TALAL, N. and DECKER, J. L. (1971). *Ann. intern. Med.*, **75**, 165.

SZTEJNBOK, M., STEWART, A., DIAMOND, H. and KAPLAN, D. (1971), *Arthr. and Rheum.*, **14**, 639.

TURK, J. L., PARKER, D. and POULTER, L. W. (1972). *Immunology*, **23**, 493.

WEINBERG, A. L. (1975). In *Progress in Immunology*, Vol. II, 5, p. 253. Ed. L. Brent and J. Holborow. North Holland Publishing Co., Amsterdam.

WEISMAN, M. and ZVAIFLER, N. (1975). *J. clin. Invest.*, **56**, 725.

WINKELSTEIN, A., MIKULLA, J. M., NANKIN, H. R., POLLOCK, B. H. and STOLZER, B. L. (1972). *J. Lab. clin. Med.*, **80**, 506.

Section C

Interrelationships between Genetic Factors, Rheumatic Diseases and Immune Responses

13

Genetic Factors, Immune Response, Complement Deficiency and Susceptibility to Inflammatory Rheumatic Diseases

Introduction

A hypothesis linking certain inflammatory rheumatic diseases and immune responses is central to the theme of this book, and much evidence has been cited in support of this concept; however, the factors initiating the immune response and leading to its persistence remain largely unknown. The difficulty in detecting initiating factors may be due to the possibility that such factors are environmental agents which do not normally induce disease, but which, in genetically susceptible individuals, may do so by subtle interaction with the immunological system. Examples of possible environmental agents include certain viruses which commonly co-exist with the mammalian species without producing any immune response or disease, but which in certain species and/or experimentally manipulated conditions, prove to be immunogenic and pathogenic (e.g. C-type viruses which are commensals in murine mammals, but which have been shown to be involved in the pathogenesis of natural or experimentally acquired autoimmune and malignant diseases in certain genetic strains of mice). Other environmental agents suspected to be involved in inducing or exacerbating immunologically mediated diseases include drugs (producing haemolytic anaemias, lupus syndromes and immune-complex nephritis) and ultraviolet solar radiation (which aggravates SLE). Obviously, the pathways involved in mediating the disease process are complex but, if immunological in nature, seem to involve specific immunological reactions to putative environmental antigens or be associated with the induction of autoimmune reactions; in both instances it can be concluded that an 'abnormal' response has followed on a 'common' exposure. It is suggested that the susceptibility to certain rheumatic diseases corresponds to this pattern, and is determined genetically.

The genetic factors altering immune responses relevant to rheumatic diseases could operate at many levels and lead to several possible models of disease susceptibility. The following are discussed in this chapter:

1. The loss of synthetic capacity of essential effector molecules of the immune response, characterized by:
    (a) immunoglobulin deficiencies, and
    (b) a range of complement deficiencies that are now being defined.

2. The development of antigen-specific responses peculiar to the individual with a particular genetic composition. Antigen-specific responses to autoantigens (e.g. rheumatoid and anti-nuclear factors in rheumatoid arthritis and SLE) and to environmental agents (e.g. streptococci in rheumatic fever) are believed to be of pathogenetic importance, but little is known of their genetic control. In guinea-pigs and mice it has proved possible to define particular genes which are related to susceptibility to thyroiditis (Vladutiu and Rose, 1971), a disease resulting from an autoimmune response to thyroid antigens. It has recently become evident that in animals and man the region on chromosomes concerned with the genetic control of immune response (IR genes) is close to the genes which code for a variety of transplantation antigens expressed on cell surface membranes, which (in man) are termed 'human leucocyte antigens' (HL-A).*

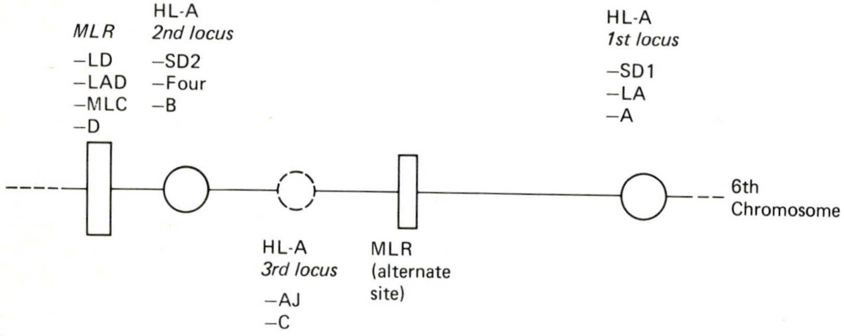

Postulated regions on the above map for genes concerned with:

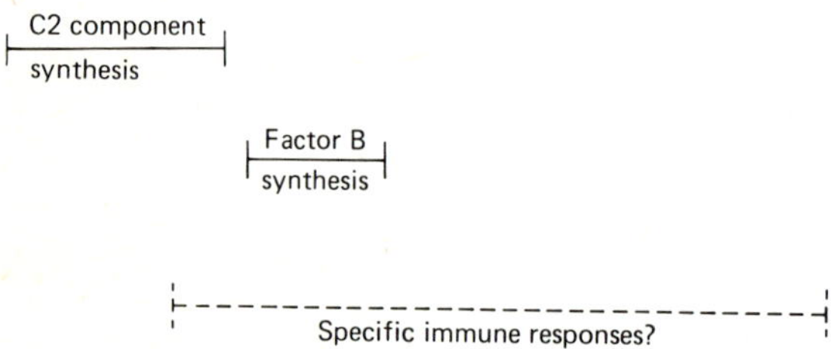

Fig. 13.1   The major histocompatibility complex in man is provisionally located on the 6th chromosome. Loci are shown which are postulated to express three HL-A* and two MLR membrane antigens; the alternative forms of nomenclature are shown. The hypothetical sites for genes controlling immune response, and C2 and factor B are believed to be close to the same region as HL-A and MLR loci.

The chromosome region is itself termed the 'major histocompatability complex' (MHC) and includes genes which control lymphocyte antigens (termed LD) which interact and stimulate allogeneic lymphocyte transformation in mixed lymphocyte reactions (MLR) (Fig. 13.1) (Jongsma et al., 1973; McDevitt and Bodmer, 1974).

* See Appendix, p. 139.

The existence of a link between IR genes and genes controlling HL-A and LD antigens allows the use of the latter as markers for genes controlling specific immune response. The initial observation on inbred laboratory animals has been followed by a description of association of HL-A types with sensitivity to ragweed pollen antigens in certain families, thus providing evidence for the association of IR genes, histocompatibility antigens and disease in man (Levine *et al.*, 1972; Blumenthal *et al.*, 1974). There is now considerable literature on the association or otherwise of histocompatibility antigens and some types of rheumatic disease, and it is possible to postulate that in these diseases such HL-A markers indicate the presence of abnormal immune responses to environmental (or intrinsic) antigens dictated by IR genes.

The concept of genetic predisposition to rheumatic diseases is not new; however, until recently, the available tools were limited to population studies with particular emphasis on twin and family studies.

Epidemiology and genetic predisposition

Epidemiologists, using family and twin studies, have sought concentrations of rheumatic diseases that might suggest a genetic predisposition. Ankylosing spondylitis has been found in one study to be 22·6 times as frequent in relatives of spondylitics as in controls, whereas, in a parallel study, rheumatoid arthritis was found 2·8 times more frequently amongst relatives of rheumatoid arthritis patients (De Blecourt *et al.*, 1961). The strong familial tendency for the development of spondylitis provided the best example of genetic predisposition in the rheumatic diseases where reliance has been placed principally on epidemiological methods. With this notable exception, the results in other rheumatic diseases (where immunological mechanisms are implicated) have been equivocal.

In patients with rheumatoid arthritis there are examples of family studies with an apparently raised concentration of affected subjects. For example, Lawrence, taking one of the more easily defined features of rheumatoid arthritis —the erosions seen on x-ray—found an increased incidence of the disease (as shown in Table 13.1) in first-degree relatives of patients with sero-positive rheumatoid disease, whilst in sero-negative patients the familial incidence was not increased (see Table 13.1) (Lawrence, 1967).

Table 13.1 Familial incidence of rheumatoid arthritis

	No. of relatives examined	No with. erosions	Expected incidence of erosive disease
Sero-positive*	342	40 (12%)	13·6 (4%)
Sero-negative	296	9 (3%)	10·7 (3.6%)

* Sheep cell agglutination test in probands.

In juvenile rheumatoid arthritis (JRA), radiological evidence of erosive disease was found four times as commonly in the female relatives when compared to age- and sex-matched controls (Ansel *et al.*, 1962). Juvenile chronic polyarthritis is a heterogeneous group of conditions, and it is not surprising that those probands who ultimately developed sacroiliitis or spondylitis (and who show a high incidence of HL-A-27) were also found to have a high incidence of relatives with sacroiliitis or ankylosing spondylitis (Edmonds *et al.*, 1974).

Some twin studies in rheumatoid arthritis have shown concordance in monozygous pairs and, to a lesser extent, in dizygous pairs; the results of other studies have not been consistent (Lawrence, 1967). The methodology involved and some of the fallacies inherent in these investigations have been reviewed and doubt expressed as to their interpretation (O'Brien, 1967). If such data are to be interpreted as showing hereditability factors, concepts of incomplete penetrance and polygenic control must be invoked. The likelihood of such genetic predisposition when compared with environmental factors is probably no more than 30–40 per cent, based on the available epidemiological data. This is similar to that which might be found in diseases in which there are clearly defined aetiological factors other than heredity; for example, chronic pulmonary tuberculosis. A similar picture exists in family and twin studies of patients with systemic lupus erythematosus. Black American females have been noted to have a threefold excess of SLE as compared with caucasian Americans; both groups have a greater incidence when in an urban rather than a rural environment, the racial differences being maintained, perhaps indicative of both genetic and environmental contributions to aetiology (Leanhardt, 1967; Siegel and Lee, 1973).

The problems involved in separating these degrees of genetic versus environmental control, stem partially from diagnostic difficulties encountered in both RA and SLE and the fact that both diseases become apparent relatively late in adult life, thus aggravating design difficulties in epidemiological surveys.

Genetic control of the non-antigen-specific immune response and rheumatic disease

IMMUNOGLOBULIN DEFICIENCY

The inherited and acquired deficiencies of immunoglobulin production are associated in approximately half of the affected individuals with a polyarthritis resembling rheumatoid arthritis and, to a much lesser degree, with dermatomyositis (Good *et al.*, 1957; Rosen and Janeway, 1966). The arthritis, which can be nodular, differs from rheumatoid disease in some respects: rheumatoid factor is absent and the disease is less destructive than the adult form of rheumatoid arthritis. A cellular basis for the synovial inflammation has been suspected, but evidence of complement consumption in joint fluids with C3 deposits in the synovial membrane without Ig or early component deposits raises the possibility of alternate pathway activation of complement (Munthe *et al.*, 1975). There is a good clinical response to gammaglobulin therapy. Whatever the relationship to adult RA, it is conceivable that the polyarthritis results from undue susceptibility to infection consequent upon immunoglobulin deficiency (although organisms are not usually found and the synovitis responds clinically to injections of immunoglobulin but not to antibiotics).

Deficiencies of individual classes of immunoglobulins may be associated with inflammatory polyarthritis; for example, IgA (Panush *et al.*, 1972; Cassidy *et al.*, 1973). A deficiency of IgA has been reported in JRA and in SLE. Whether these class deficiencies are inherited or acquired is not established. In contrast, deficiency of IgG subclasses is associated not with predisposition to connective tissue diseases but with pyogenic pulmonary infections (Schur *et al.*, 1970).

COMPLEMENT COMPONENT DEFICIENCIES

Individual components of the complement enzyme system have been found to be deficient, or partially so, in the sera of several family groups. Some of the members of these groups have rheumatic diseases (Table 13.2), inheritance of the com-

Table 13.2   Complement component deficiencies and rheumatic diseases

Component deficiency	Associated disease	Reference
C1r	SLE	Moncado *et al.*, 1972
		Day *et al.*, 1972
		Pickering *et al.*, 1970
C1s	Infection, arthralgias and SLE	Pondman *et al*, 1968
C1 INH	Angioedema with SLE	Kohler *et al.*, 1974
C4	SLE	Hauptmann *et al.*, 1974
C2	Monoarthritis	Cooper *et al.*, 1968
	SLE	Agnello *et al.*, 1972
		Day *et al.*, 1973
		Osterland *et al.*, 1975
	Discoid LE	Osterland *et al.*, 1975
	Dermatomyositis	Leddy *et al.*, 1975
	Anaphylactoid purpura	Susman *et al.*, 1973
C5	SLE	Rosenfeld & Leddy, 1974

ponent deficiency being autosomal dominant in those identified so far. The syndromes resembling systemic lupus erythematosus found in these patients have not been entirely typical; anti-nuclear antibodies, for example, are not found to the same extent as in SLE patients.

The component deficiencies detected most commonly so far are those which make up the early part of the classical pathway, the most common deficiency being that of C2 complement component. Complement deficiency in individuals heterozygous for the gene controlling the synthesis of complement component (and therefore with 30–60 per cent of the normal levels of the particular protein), does not always seem to be associated with disease. This is particularly true for C2, where the families described initially were generally asymptomatic (Ruddy *et al.*, 1970).

Reports published to date on C2 deficiency have concentrated on family studies. Although the incidence of C2 deficiency in rheumatic disease populations is not known, preliminary reports suggest that there is an increased concentration of heterozygous-deficient individuals amongst JRA and SLE patients (Schur, personal communication).

There are limited data available on the incidence of hypocomplementaemia, either inherited or acquired, in a general population. Those studies that are available suggest an incidence of between 0·1 and 0·01 per cent (Von Hassig *et al.*, 1964; Stratton, 1974). Von Hassig *et al.* found 14 complement-deficient subjects when examining the sera of 41,083 recruits to the Swiss army, while Stratton was able to find 1 complement-deficient person examining 10,000 sera from blood bank donors and this person was deficient in C2. These figures probably relate to homozygous deficiencies only; an estimated incidence of heterozygous deficiency based on these figures might be in the order of 1 in 50 to 1 in 100 for C2.

The recently described association between histocompatibility antigens HL-A-10 and/or W18 and C2 deficiency provides a tool for the study of the epidemiology of complement deficiency. These particular antigens, HL-A-10/W18, have not been found more commonly in SLE than in a general population, a finding consistent with the probable incidence of C2 deficiency in SLE; not all subjects with this haplotype are C2 deficient.

Loci for control of other complement components are likely to be found if animal models can be translated to human studies (Fu *et al.*, 1974; Ferreira and Nussenzweig, 1975; Gibson *et al.*, 1975); indeed Allen has recently reported the association of HL-A-12 with one of the allotypes of factor B (GBG) of the alternate pathway (Allen, 1974).

Markers for possible antigen-specific immune response genes and rheumatic disease

It would seem that where a process of randomization of the genetic pool has not occurred and particular HL-A antigens are linked to particular immune response genes, the HL-A antigens can be used indirectly as markers for immunologically mediated disease. The histocompatibility antigens in man closest to the suggested site for the immune response genes are those of the second series HL-A types and the mixed lymphocyte reaction (MLR) locus. Evidence is also accumulating for the existence of a third HL-A site (SD3 or AJ) close to the second series site, the definition of which is incomplete (see Fig. 13.1).

There is evidence that the histocompatibility complex is to be found on the 6th autosomal chromosome in a manner analogous to the H_2 loci on the 17th chromosome of the mouse. The lack of readily available antisera for use in the definition of the MLR loci (as are available for the HL-A antigens) is a limiting factor, but in ankylosing spondylitis there is a striking association between an HL-A type and a clinical entity. Associations between disease and MLR loci are being recognized (e.g. for multiple sclerosis; Jersild *et al.*, 1974).

The demonstration of an association between disease and histocompatibility (HL-A) antigens could therefore provide evidence for the existence of genetic control, and by inference suggests an immune basis for disease, assuming IR genes and HL-A antigens are as closely related in man as is currently believed.

HL-A-27 SPONDYLITIS

The association between tissue type HL-A-27 and ankylosing spondylitis represents the closest associations known between a given HL-A antigen and disease or at least part of its pathology (Brewerton *et al.*, 1973; Schlosstein *et al.*, 1973). The link between HL-A-27 and disease seems to be directed particularly towards sacroiliitis, whether this be part of ankylosing spondylitis, Reiter's syndrome, psoriatic arthritis or the arthropathies associated with bowel disease. While the proportion of spondylitis with HL-A-27 may be greater than 90 per cent over all, it was estimated that 5 per cent or less of HL-A-27 individuals will have clinical evidence of spondylitis, although a higher incidence may in fact be the case (Calin and Fries, 1975).

The genetic abnormality represents only predisposition to disease; this will not develop unless the individual meets some as yet unidentified environmental hazard. Explanations other than the presence of IR genes have been suggested to explain the link between HL-A antigens and disease. These alternative hypotheses include antigenic cross-reaction between a presumed virus and HL-A antigens, and adaptation of host proteins (including HL-A antigens) to provide membranes for a possible pathogen. The generally defined lack of an aetiological agent, or a readily measurable gene product, makes the testing of any hypothesis difficult for the HL-A-27 spondylitis link. The specific agents so far identified in HL-A-27-associated spondylitis are *Yersinia enterocolitica* reported from Scandinavia, and those patients with Reiter's syndrome associated with a Salmonella or Shigella gastrointestinal infection. Aho *et al.* (1974) have reported an incidence of HL-A-27 in 43 of 49 patients with Yersinia arthritis; this link might prove to be of interest in investigating the association between the specific antigen, arthritis and HL-A-27.

A lower level of lymphocyte transformation has been reported to Yersinia-derived antigens in HL-A-27 individuals, compared with the response to PHA or Candida (Nibkin *et al.*, 1975).

It is evident in a review of two family studies that an HL-A-27-linked gene is not the sole determinant of predisposition to spondylitis. One of the family studies reported from Holland involved a non-HL-A-27 father with spondylitis, born from a marriage between first cousins, whose children acquired HL-A-27 from their mother. The children with HL-A-27 developed spondylitis, suggesting that two genes are required, the father being homozygous for the non-HL-A-27-linked gene and the children with disease being heterozygous for both genes. By inference, the homozygous state of the non-HL-A-27-linked gene can give disease susceptibility and for the heterozygous state both genes are required.

OTHER RHEUMATIC DISEASES

Tissue type antigen associations have been investigated in other inflammatory rheumatic diseases including juvenile polyarthritis (JRA), rheumatoid arthritis and systemic lupus erythematosus. In JRA the variable degree in which HL-A-27 is found probably reflects the differing proportions of patients with ankylosing spondylitis who present initially in a manner clinically indistinguishable from JRA, and the length of follow-up in the reported surveys. In rheumatoid arthritis abnormal concentrations of antigens have not been defined and in SLE several different antigens have been reported present in increased frequency (Table 13.3). Racial differences in HL-A types may account for some of these variations.

Table 13.3   HL-A tissue typing in systemic lupus erythematosus

Antigen		Patients*	Controls	Reference
HL-A-5	Caucasian	24% (42)	11% (886)	Nies *et al.*, 1974
	Negroid	23% (40)	5% (120)	
HL-A-8	Caucasian	36% (40)	16% (82)	Grumet *et al.*, 1971
W15		36% (40)	10% (82)	
W15	—	21% (24)	—	Waters & Walford, 1971
HL-A-13	Negroid	15% (40)	0% (40)	Arnett *et al.*, 1972
W19	Negroid	52% (40)	7% (40)	Stastny, 1972
W5	Negroid	2x as frequent as in controls		

* The percentage figure is the prevalence of the HL-A type in the sample tested; the figure in parentheses refers to the number of individuals tested.

Epidemiological studies of these diseases do not suggest as homogeneous a degree of genetic control as exists in ankylosing spondylitis and, therefore, even if there are particular IR genes involved, HL-A linkage will be more difficult to determine. The reported incidence of IgA and C2 deficiency in SLE and the diverse precipitating factors, ranging from drugs to sunlight, suggests heterogeneity of both genetic and environmental factors which is reflected in the range of HL-A type reported in SLE. The search for genetic markers is further complicated in that it is apparent that HL-A loci represent only part of the histocompatibility complex, the MLR locus or loci being seemingly independent of the HL-A system. MLR responses have been measured between lymphocytes from patients with rheumatoid arthritis and a reduced degree of responsiveness was found (Astorga and Williams, 1969) as shown in Table 13.4.

Table 13.4

Cell source	Pairs tested	No stimulation
RA vs RA*	22	14/22
RA vs normal*	22	6/22
Normal vs RA*	22	3/22

* Mitomycin-treated.

In a more recent study Stastny (1974) has found a markedly increased prevalence of two defined MLR loci in the majority of rheumatoid patients. The evidence so far available suggests that if markers are to be identified in RA and JRA the linkage is more likely to be with MLR or other HL-A antigens rather than those of the first or second series.

Conclusions

The extent to which genetic factors either mediating immunodeficiency or controlling the direction of the immune response, can predispose individuals to rheumatic diseases is not understood. The known protein deficiencies appear to be more common than anticipated but have been found in only a minority of patients. The parallel studies identifying histocompatibility antigen associations may point towards the polygenic nature of the genetic control, although the mechanism whereby this brings about disease is also very incompletely understood.

References

AGNELLO, V., DE BRACCO, M. M. E. and KUNKEL, H. G. (1972). *J. Immunol.*, **108**, 837.

AHO, K., AHVONEN, P. LASSUS, A., SIEVERS, K. and TIILIKAINER, A. (1974). *Arthr. and Rheum*, **17**, 521.

ALLEN, F. H. (1974). *Vox Sang. (Basel)*, **27**, 382.

ANSELL, B. M., BYWATERS, E. G. L. and LAWRENCE, J. S. (1962). *Ann. rheum. Dis.*, **21**, 243.

ARNETT, F. C., BIAS, W. B. and SHULMAN, L. E. (1972). *Arthr. and Rheum.*, **15**, 428.

ASTORGA, G. P. and WILLIAMS, R. C., Jr. (1969). *Arthr. and Rheum.*, **12**, 547.

BLUMENTHAL, M. N., AMOS, D. B., NOREEN, H., MENDELL, N. R. and YUNIS, E. J. (1974). *Science*, **184**, 1301.

BREWERTON, D. A., CAFFREY, M., HART, F. D., JAMES, D. C. O., NICHOLLS, A. and STURROCK, R. D. (1973). *Lancet*, **1**, 904.

CALIN, A. and FRIES, J. R. (1975). *New Engl. J. Med.*, **293**, 835.

CASSIDY, J. T., PETTY, R. E. and SULLIVAN, D. B. (1973). *J. clin. Invest.*, **52**, 1931.

COOPER, N. R., TEN BENSEL, R. and KOHLER, P. F. (1968). *J. Immonul.*, **101**, 1176.

DAY, N. K., GEIGER, H., STROUD, R., DE BRACCO, M., MONCADO, B., WINDHORST, D. and GOOD, R. A. (1972). *J. clin. Invest.*, **51**, 1102.

DAY, N. K., GEIGER, H., MCLEAN, R., MICHAEL, A. and GOOD, R. A. (1973). *J. clin. Invest.*, **52**, 160.

DE BLECOURT, J. J., POLMAN, A. and DE BLECOURT-MEINDERSMA, T. (1961). *Ann. rheum. Dis.*, **20**, 21.

EDMONDS, J., MORRIS, R. I., METZGER, A. L., BLUESTONE, R., TERASAKI, P. I., ANSELL, B. and BYWATERS, E. G. L. (1974). *Ann. rheum. Dis.*, **33**, 289.

FERREIRA, A. and NUSSENZWEIG, V. (1975). *J. exp. Med.*, **141**, 513.

FU, S. M., KUNKEL, H. G., BRUSMAN, H. P., ALLEN, F. H., Jr. and FOTINO, M. (1974). *J. exp. Med.*, **140**, 1108.

GIBSON, D., GLASS, D. N., CARPENTER, C. B. and SCHUR, P. H. (1975). *Arthr. and Rheum.* (in press) (abstr.).

GOOD, R. A., ROTSTEIN, J. and MAZZITELLO, W. F. (1957). *J. Lab. clin. Med.*, **49**, 343.

GRUMET, F. C., COOKELL, A. and BODMER, J. G. (1971). *New Engl. J. Med.*, **285**, 193.

HAUPTMANN, G., GROSSHANS, E. and REID, E. (1974). *Ann. Derm. Syph. (Paris)*, **101**, 479.

JERSILD, C., HANSEN, G. S., SVEJGAARD, A., FOG, T., THOMSEN, M. and DUPONT, B. (1974). *Lancet*, **2**, 1221.

JONGSMA, A., VAN SOMERN, H., WESTERVELD, A., HAGEMEIJER, A. and PEARSON, P. (1973). *Hum. Genet.*, **20**, 195.

KOHLER, P. F., PERCY, J., CAMPION, W. M. and SMYTH, C. J. (1974). *Amer. J. Med.*, **56**, 406.

LAWRENCE, J. S. (1967). *Clin. exp. Immunol.*, **2**, 769.

LEANHARDT, E. T. G. (1967). *Clin. exp. Immunol.*, **2**, 243.

LEDDY, J. P., GRIGGS, R. C., KLEMPERER, M. R. and FRANK, M. M. (1975). *Amer. J. Med.*, **58**, 83.

LEVINE, B. B., STEMBER, R. H. and FOTINO, M. (1972). *Science*, **178**, 1201.

MCDEVITT, H. O. and BODMER, W. F. (1974). *Lancet*, **1**, 1269.

MONCADO, B., DAY, N. K. B., GOOD, R. A. and WINDHORST, D. B. (1972). *New Engl. J. Med.*, **286**, 689.

MUNTHE, E., HOYERALL, H. M., FROLAND, S. S., MELLBYE, O. J., KASS, E. and NATVIG, J. B. (1975). *Rheumatology*, **6**, 43.

NIBKIN, B., BREWERTON, D. A., BYROM, N., JAMES, D. C. O., MALKA, S., MCLEOD, L., SLATER, L., WARREN, R. E. and HOBBS, J. R. (1975). *Ann. rheum. Dis.*, **34**, 49.

NIES, H. M., BROWN, J. C., DUBOIS, E. L., QUISMORIO, F. P., FRIOU, G. J. and TERASAKI, P. I. (1974). *Arthr. and Rheum.*, **17**, 397.

O'BRIEN, W. M. (1967). *Clin. exp. Immunol.*, **2**, 785.

OSTERLAND, C. K., ESPINOZA, L., PARKER, L. P., and SCHUR, P. H. (1975). *Ann. intern. Med.*, **82**, 32.

PANUSH, R. S., BIANCO, N. E., SCHUR, P. H., ROCKLIN, R. E., DAVID, J. R. and STILLMAN, J. S. (1972). *Clin, exp. Immunol.*, **10**, 103.

PICKERING, R. J., NAFF, G. B., STROUD, R. M., GOOD, R. A. and GEWURZ, H. (1970). *J. exp. Med.*, **131**, 803.

PONDMAN, K. W., STOOP, J. W., CORMANE, R. H. and HANNEMA, A. J. (1968). *J. Immunol.*, **101**, 811 (abstr.).

ROSEN, F. S. and JANEWAY, C. A. (1966). *New Engl. J. Med.*, **275**, 709.

ROSENFELD, S. I. and LEDDY, J. P. (1974). *J. clin. Invest.*, **53**, 67a (abstr.).

RUDDY, S., KLEMPERER, M. R., ROSEN, F. S., AUSTEN, K. F. and KUMATE, J. (1970). *Immunology*, **18**, 943.

SCHLOSSTEIN, L., TERASAKI, P. I., BLUESTONE, R. and PEARSON, C. M. (1973). *New Engl. J. Med.*, **288**, 704.

SCHUR, P. H., BOREL, H., GELFAND, E. W., ALPER, C. A. and ROSEN, F. S. (1970). *New Engl. J. Med.*, **283**, 631.

SIEFEL, M. and LEE, S. L. (1973). *Semin. Arthritis Rheum.*, **3**, 1.

STASTNY, P. (1972). *Arthr. and Rheum.*, **15**, 455.

STASTNY, P. (1974). *Tissue Antigens*, **4**, 571.

STRATTON, F., quoted in LACHMANN, P. J. (1974). *Boll. 1st sieroter. Milan*, **53**, 195 (suppl.).

SUSSMAN, M., JONES, J. H., ALMEIDA, J. D. and LACHMANN, P. J. (1973). *Clin. exp. Immunol.*, **14**, 531.

VLADUTIU, A. O. and ROSE, N. R. (1971). *Science*, **174**, 1137.

VON HASSIG, A., BOREL, J. F., AMMANN, P., THORII, M. and BUTLER, R. (1964). *Pathol. Microbiol.*, **27**, 542.

WATERS, K. P. and WALFORD, R. L. (1971). *Tissue Antigens*, **1**, 68.

Appendix

New* and previous terminologies for major histocompatibility region antigens (HLA specificities) determined by serological or mixed leucocyte culture tests

A locus†		B locus		C locus	
New	Previous	New	Previous	New	Previous
HLA-A1	HL-A1	HLA-B5	HL-A5	HLA-CW1	T1
HLA-A2	HL-A2	HLA-B7	HL-A7	HLA-CW2	T2
HLA-A3	HL-A3	HLA-B8	HL-A8	HLA-CW3	T3
HLA-A9	HL-A9	HLA-B12	HL-A12	HLA-CW4	T4
HLA-A10	HL-A10	HLA-B13	HL-A13	HLA-CW5	T5
HLA-A11	HL-A11	HLA-B14	W14		
HLA-A28	W28	HLA-B18	W18		
HLA-A29	W29	HLA-B27	W27		
HLA-AW23	W23	HLA-BW15	W15		
HLA-AW24	W24	HLA-BW16	W16		
HLA-AW25	W25	HLA-BW17	W17		
HLA-AW26	W26	HLA-BW21	W21	D locus	
HLA-AW30	W30	HLA-BW22	W22		
HLA-AW31	W31	HLA-BW35	W5	HLA-DW1	LD 101
HLA-AW32	W32	HLA-BW37	TY	HLA-DW2	LD 102
HLA-AW33	W19.6	HLA-BW38	W16.1	HLA-DW3	LD 103
HLA-AW34	Malay 2	HLA-BW39	W16.2	HLA-DW4	LD 104
HLA-AW36	MO	HLA-BW40	W10	HLA-DW5	LD 105
HLA-AW43	BK	HLA-BW41	Sabell	HLA-DW6	LD 106
		HLA-BW42	MWA		

† WHO-IUIS terminology committee nomenclature for factors of the HL-A system.
* See Fig. 13.1 for location on chromosone 6 and alternative designations.

Index

agammaglobulinaemia 8, 18, 66, 132–3
'alternate pathway' complement activa-
    tion 41, 42, 60, 73, 80
ankylosing spondylitis 7, 18, 132, 134–5
antibodies 98–9
    anti-chondrocyte 28
    anti-collagen 29
    anti-DNA 30–3, 74, 77, 78, 79, 80
    anti-DNA-histone 30–2
    anti-DS-DNA 30–2, 74, 79, 90
    anti-ENA 30–2, 79
    anti-globulin (*see* rheumatoid factors)
    anti-lymphocyte 45, 47 (*also see*
        lymphocytotoxic antibodies)
    anti-nuclear (ANA) 9, 10, 29–33, 79,
        99
        detection by immunofluorescence
            30
        heterogeneity 33
        staining patterns 30
    anti-nucleolar components 32
    anti-proteoglycans 28, 101
    anti-RNA 30–2, 83
    anti-receptor (motor-end plate) 99
    anti-SS-DNA 31–2, 74, 79, 85, 90
    anti-skeletal muscle 96, 97, 98
    anti-Sm 32
    clinical significance to nuclear and
        cytoplasmic antigens 31
    detection as immune complexes 43
    lymphocytotoxic 81, 84, 99
    non-organ specific 23
    organ-specific 23
    phagocytosed 39
    production 5
    synthesized 39, 40
    thymus 98
antigen(s)
    arterial extract 34, 117
    Australia 109–10, 116
    cytoplasmic 31
    DNA 34, 35, 73, 74, 79
    detection 43
    hypersensitivity reactions to 5–7
    IgG 23–8, 34

IgM 34
    muscle 34, 98
    Mycoplasma 35, 68
    nuclear 31
    salivary gland 34, 90
    synovial cell line 34, 67–8
    synovial membrane 34
    T-cell-specific 46
antigenic sites on IgG 24
antigen-specific responses 4–5, 130
anti-globulin factors 23–4 (*also see* rheu-
    matoid factors)
arteritis
    giant cell 114, 117
    polyarteritis nodosa 116
    vasculitis, and 115
Arthus phenomenon 14
Arthus reaction 16, 17, 109
Australia antigen 109–10, 116
autoantibody 9, 23–33
autoantigen(s)
    cellular immunity to 33–5
    immune reactions to 23–35
autoimmunity 8–12

B cells 4, 5, 8–12, 45–7, 62–5, 81, 90
Behcet's syndrome 114, 118
biopsy
    excision 38
    percutaneous 38
    'punch' needle 38

C3 receptor 46, 47
C3 rosette 39, 47
CH_{50} 41
cell(s)
    adherence to glass 46, 48
    adherence to Nylon 46, 48
    cytotoxicity 19–21, 46
cellular immunity
    antigens and 4–5
    autoantigens, to 33–5
    DNA, to 35
    IgG, to 33, 34, 68
    pathogenesis, connective tissue
        disease 18–21

cellular immunity—*cont.*
  tests 44–9
  thymus-dependent lymphocytes 4, 7,
    19
central nervous system and systemic
  lupus erythematosus 75–6
chondrocyte(s)
  antibody to 28
  necrosis 28
chromatography 43
chronic discoid lupus erythematosus
  (CDLE) 84–5
  clinical features 84
  systemic lupus erythematosus and 84–
    85
'classical pathway' complement activation 41, 42, 60, 73, 80
collagen, antibodies to 29
columns
  antibody-coated 48
  Nylon-fibre 48
complement 6–7, 40–2, 60, 79–81
  anaphlytoxin activity 17
  binding complexes to 16, 17, 43
  Clq 26, 27, 29, 43, 58, 73, 74, 80
  cerebrospinal fluid, in 76,
  chemotactic activity 17
  component deficiencies 133
    family studies 133
    incidence 133–4
  cytolysis 17
  decrease 41–2
  deposition 42
  inactivation products 42, 60
  rheumatoid arthritis, and 60
  rheumatoid factor, binding to 25
  role in tissue injury 16–17
  sequential activation 41
  skin in 76, 85
  systemic lupus erythematosus and
    73–5, 79–81
  turnover 59, 60
cryoprecipitates 43, 80
cytoplasm, staining 48
cytostatic drugs 121–4
  complications 122, 123
  dermatomyositis 123
  polymyositis 123
  rheumatoid arthritis 121
  systemic lupus erythematosus 121–3
    studies 122
  vasculitis 121
  Wegener's granulomatosis 123

cytotoxicity
  cell-mediated 19–20, 43, 49, 65, 97
  K cell 6, 20, 46, 49
  mononuclear cell 17, 20, 21

DNA (*see* antibodies, to, and antigen(s))
  homologous sequences with RNA 84
delayed hypersensitivity 7, 34, 46, 49,
  64, 81–2
dermatomyositis 95, 97, 115
  and cytostatic drugs 123
drug-induced lupus erythematosus 85–6

E rosette 39, 46, 47, 62, 63, 81, 90, 91
EA rosette 39, 46, 48, 62, 63
EAC rosette 39, 46, 47, 62, 81
ENA (extractable nuclear antigen), antibody to 30, 31, 32, 79
E-Rc (*see* E rosette)
environmental factors 129, 132, 136
epidemiology 131–2
extractable nuclear antigen (ENA), antibody to (*see* ENA)

Fab fragments 27, 28
  fluorescein-conjugated, anti-Ig 47, 63
Farr binding assay 30–1, 79
Fc receptors 44–5, 46, 48, 63
fresh tissue studies 38
  source of material 38

genetic factors 7, 129–37
  antigen-specific response 130–1, 134–
    135
  complement deficiencies 129, 133, 134
  epidemiology 131–2
  immunoglobulin deficiencies 129
giant cell arteritis 114, 117
glomerular basement membrane (GBM)
  15, 73, 75
Gm markers 24

HL-A (human leucocyte antigen) 130–1
  markers, as 134
  racial differences 135, 136
  spondylitis, and 7–8, 134–5
  systemic lupus erythematosus and
    135, 136
  terminology (old and new) 139
haemolytic activity of complement 41,
  42
heavy chain determinants 24
  on lymphocytes 91

helper effect 4, 8
Henoch-Schönlein purpura 114, 118
hepatitis B infections 109–10, 116
heterogeneity, human lymphoid cells 44
histamine release 43
homogenous staining 30
homoreactants 27
  antibody 28
human leucocyte antigen (*see* HL-A)
humoral immunity, abnormalities 10
hypersensitivity, delayed (*see* delayed
    hypersensitivity)
hypersensitivity reactions
  type I 5–6
  type II 6, 23
  type III 6–7, 18, 23
  type IV 7, 18

idiotypic specificity 25, 74
Ig, surface 44, 45, 46, 47 (*also see* B cells)
IgG
  aggregated 24, 33, 34
  papain-treated 27
  reactions to 24, 33
IgG-coated latex agglutination inhibi-
    tion 43
immune complex(es)
  circulating 14–16, 58–9
    measurement 42–4
  clearance 5, 15, 16, 75
  complement, and 16–17, 41, 43
  DNA-anti-DNA 79–80
  deposition 14–16
  formation 14–15
  hypersensitivity (Type III) reactions
    6–7
  localization 15
  persistence 15
  phagocytosis 17, 75
  rheumatoid 57–9
  systemic lupus erythematosus 79–81
  tissue damage, and 14–17
  vasculitis and 113
immune response 3–12, 129
  biological aspects 3–12
  cell-mediated, impairment of 64, 66–
    67, 81–2, 91
  extrinsic antigens, to 64, 66, 67–8, 81–
    84
  factors altering 129–30
  factors initiating 129
  genetic control 7–8, 130, 132, 134–6
  induction 4–5

inflammatory rheumatic diseases and
    129
  mechanisms 3–4
immune status 64–7
  in juvenile rheumatoid arthritis 66–7
  in rheumatoid arthritis 64–6
  in systemic lupus erythematosus 81–2
immunochemistry 40
immunodeficiency
  of IgA 66, 133
  of IgG 8, 18, 66, 132–3
immunofluorescent staining 39
immunofluorescent tests 29–31
immunoglobulin deficiency (*see*
    immunodeficiency)
immunological methods 38–49
immunoregulation 10, 54, 124
immunostimulation 124
immunosuppression 120–1
  antigen-antibody complexes, plasma-
    pheresis of 120
  drugs and 120, 121, 124
  lymphocytes, removal of 120
infections
  arthritis and 103–9
    bacteria 68, 103, 104, 105
    classification 103–5
    hepatitis B infections 109–10
    meningococcal arthritis 109
    mycoplasma 68, 105
    rheumatic fever 106–9
    viruses 103, 104, 105
  immune reactions to 67–8
inflammatory rheumatic diseases
  environmental factors 129
  genetic factors 129–34
  immune responses and 129
inflammatory vascular disease, classi-
    fication 114

joint
  diagram 54
  infections 103–6
  normal 53
  rheumatoid arthritis 53–5
  systemic lupus erythematosus 71–2
juvenile rheumatoid arthritis 66–7, 131–
    132, 133, 135

kidney and experimentally induced
    immune complex disease 14–16
kidney and systemic lupus
    erythematosus 72–5, 79, 80, 121–2

LE cell(s) 33
  phenomenon 29, 52
leucocyte migration test 34, 35, 44, 68,
    100
liver and systemic lupus erythematosus
    77
liver disease and DNA antibodies 31
lung and systemic lupus erythematosus
    77
lymphocyte(s) 3, 4, 7, 18, 19, 20, 21
  activation 19, 20
  autoimmunity, and 8–12
  B (*see* B cells)
  cell surface characteristics 45–9
  cytotoxicity tests 34, 49
  function tests 45
  incubation 40, 45
  'null' cells 64
  rheumatoid synovial membranes, in
      57, 62
  sensitized 19, 40, 97
  subpopulations 44–7
    rheumatoid arthritis, in 62–4
    systemic lupus erythematosus, in
        81
  suppressor 5, 11–12
  T (*see* T cells)
  transformation 34, 35, 44, 45, 46, 49,
      64, 65, 82, 91, 97, 101
  synovial fluid, in 65
lymphoid cells, classifications 45–9
lymphokine(s) 4, 7, 18, 19, 21, 44, 57
  production 46, 49
  synthesis 40, 57
lymphoproliferative disorders, Sjögren's
    syndrome and 92
lymphotoxin 19, 34
lysosomal enzymes 17, 28, 57

MIF (migration inhibition factor) 7, 34,
    44, 46, 49
MLR (mixed leucocyte reaction) 46, 49,
    130, 134, 136
macrophage(s) 4, 5, 17, 20, 21, 45, 46,
    47, 48, 58
  guinea-pig 43 (*also see* MIF)
  specific macrophage arming factor
      (SMAF) 20
major histocompatibility complex
    (MHC) 130–1, 134
meningococcal arthritis 109
microbial immunity 106
microscopy 39

electron 39, 43, 73
  light 39
migration inhibition factor (*see* MIF)
mixed connective tissue disease 32
monocyte (*see* macrophage)
myasthenia gravis 94–100
  cellular immunity 99, 100
  clinical features 95
  electromyographic studies 95
  immunology 98–100
  pathology 95
  polymyositis and 95, 96
  thymic factors 99–100
  thyrotoxicosis and 94
Mycoplasma antigens 35, 68

neoplastic disease and polymyositis, 97–
    98
nodules 59
'non-self', 3
nuclear staining 30
nucleolar components, antibody to 32
nucleolar staining 30
'null' cells 64

opsonin 17, 20

pepsin agglutinators 27
periarteritis nodosa (*see* polyarteritis
    nodosa)
peripheral (membranous) staining 30
platelet aggregation 43
polyarteritis nodosa 114–16
  aetiology 116
  Australia antigen 116
  clinical features 116
  immune complexes 116
  necrotizing arteritis 116
polymyositis 94–100
  clinical features 94
  cytostatic drugs 123
  electromyographic study 95
  immunodeficiency and 97–8
  immunology 96–8
    autoantibody 96
    cellular hypersensitivity 97
    experimental models 97
    immune complexes 97
  myasthenia gravis and 95, 96, 100
  neoplastic disease and 97–8
  pathology 94–6
    type α 94
    type β 95
    type γ 95

precipitation
  double-antibody 43
  in gel 31, 33, 43
  polyethylene glycol (PEG) 43
  salt 43
prostaglandin 21, 57
proteoglycans 28, 101
  antibody to 28, 101
  cellular hypersensitivity to 101
pulseless (Takayashu's) disease 101,
    114, 117

RNA 30, 79, 83, 84
  antibody to 31, 32
Raji cell assay 43
relapsing polychondritis 101
reverse endocytosis 17
rheumatic fever 106–9
  cardiac lesions 107–8
  clinical features 107
  cross-reacting antibodies 108–9
  immunofluorescent staining 108
  streptococci, and 106, 107, 108
  tissue lesions 107–8
rheumatoid arthritis 53–68
  antibody responses 66
  antinuclear antibodies, in 30, 31
  cellular immunity 61–6, 68
  cytostatic drugs 121
  drug-induced lupus erythematosus
    and 85
  familial incidence of rheumatic
    disease 131–3
  immune mechanisms of inflammation
    53
  immunity, cellular v/s humoral 61–2
  infection, role of 67–8
  lympho-cytotoxin 66
  Mycoplasma and 68
  nodules 59
  pathogenesis 53–5
  polyarteritis nodosa and 116
  rubella and 68
  Sjögren's syndrome and 90–1
  synovial fluid in 68
  transfer factor 124
  vasculitis and 113, 115
  virus infection 67–8
rheumatoid factors 10, 23–7, 57, 58, 61,
    74, 78, 80, 90
  agglutination reactions 26, 61
  antigenic sites 24
  clinical significance 26–7

  definition 24
  heterogeneity 25–6
  'hidden', 25
  IgA 25
  IgG 25, 26, 27, 61
  IgG and 24
  IgG-anti-IgG complex formation 25,
    57
  IgM and 25–7, 61
  nature 23
  occurrence 23
  Sjögren's syndrome and 90
  systemic lupus erythematosus and 74,
    78, 80

SLE (systemic lupus erythematosus),
    71–86
  aetiology 71, 82–4, 129, 133
  autoimmune serological phenomena
    29–33, 78–9
  central nervous system involvement
    75–6
  chronic discoid lupus erythematosus
    (CDLE) 84–5
  clinical features 71
  complement 73–5, 133–4
  cytostatic drugs 121–3
  DNA antibodies 30, 31–2, 33, 79
  HL-A typing, in 134, 136
  haematological abnormalities in 78
  immune complexes 74, 79–80
  immune status 81–2
  infection, role of 82–4
  joint involvement 71–2
  kidney involvement 33, 72–5, 79,
    80
  liver involvement 77
  lung involvement 77
  lymphocyte subpopulations 81
  phagocytic activity and 75
  RNA 79, 83
  rheumatoid factor 74, 78, 80
  skin involvement 76
  synovial fluid 72
  syphilis, serological tests for, and 79
  vascular disease 77
  vasculitis and 115
  virus infection 82–4
scleroderma, antinuclear antibodies and
    30, 31, 32
'self' 3
sheep erythrocyte rosettes (*see* T cells)
sicca syndrome 89

Sjögren's syndrome 89–92
  antinuclear antibodies 90
  autoantibodies 90–1
  biopsy 89–90
  cell-mediated immunity 91
  clinical features 89
  immunopathology 89–90
  lymphocyte function 91
  lymphoproliferative disorders and 92
  peripheral blood lymphocytes 91
  rheumatoid arthritis and 90–1
  rheumatoid factor 90
  salivary duct cell antibody 90
  virus induction 92
Sm, antibody to 31, 32
specific macrophage arming factor
      (SMAF) 20
speckled staining of antinuclear anti-
      body 30
surface complement (C3) receptor (*see*
      EAC rosette)
surface immunoglobulin (*see* B cells)
synovial cells, reactions to 33–5, 68
synovial fluid 57–8, 62
  complexes 25
  in systemic lupus erythematosus 72
synovial membrane 55, 57–8
  complement 60
  immune complexes, in 57
  microscopic appearance 55–6
  rheumatoid, extract 35
  synthesis of biologically active
      molecules 57
  systemic lupus erythematosus (*see*
      SLE)
  tissue culture, of 40, 57

T cell(s)
  antisera against 47
  E (E-Rc) rosette, for detection of 39,
      46, 47
  immune response, and 4–5, 7, 19
  rheumatoid arthritis, and 62, 63
  Sjögren's syndrome, and 90, 91
  suppressor cell activity of 11–12
  systemic lupus erythematosus 81
  tolerance 8–10
      bypass or loss, 8–11
Takayashu's (pulseless) disease 101,
      114, 117
therapeutic implications 120–4

thymic hormone 99–100
tissue culture 40
tissue injury
  cell-mediated 18–21
      mechanisms 19–20
      pathogenesis 18–19
  cellular damage 13
  complement, role of 16–17
  immune complex mediated 6–7, 14–
      17
  lysosomal enzymes 17, 28, 57
  matrix damage 14
  mechanisms 13–21
  pathogenesis 15–16
  vascular damage 13, 112–13
tolerance 3, 4, 8–11
transfer factors 44, 124

ultracentrifugation
  analytical 42, 43, 58
  density gradient 43

vascular disease and systemic lupus
      erythematosus 77, 115
vascular permeability 13, 15, 17, 112
vasculitis 13, 59, 112–15
  classification 113, 114
  clinical features 112
  cytostatic drugs 121
  dermatomyositis 115
  immune complexes 113
  mycoplasma 118
  necrotizing arteritis 115
  pathogenesis 113
  rheumatoid arthritis and 113, 115
  scleroderma and 115
  systemic lupus erythematosus and 115
virus, hepatitis B (Australia antigen)
      109–10, 116
virus infection 8–10, 103–6, 109–10, 116
  oncorna 83, 84
  rheumatoid arthritis 67–8
  systemic lupus erythematosus 82–4

Wegener's granulomatosis 114, 117–18,
      123
  aetiology 118
  clinical features 117
  cytostatic drugs 123
  pathology 117